A Moder
Guide to
Dynamic Dating

Sarah Ivens is Assistant Editor of the *Sunday Mirror*'s *M Celebs* magazine and has written for *Marie Claire, Tatler, Daily Mail, News of the World* and *GQ*. Sarah is married and lives in East London.

Sarah's first book was *A Modern Girl's Guide to Getting Hitched* (Piatkus, 2002).

A Modern Girl's Guide to Dynamic Dating

How to play and win the game of love

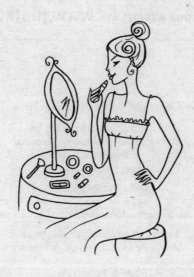

S A R A H   I V E N S

PIATKUS

First published in 2003 by
Judy Piatkus (Publishers) Limited
5 Windmill Street
London W1T 2JA

e-mail: info@piatkus.co.uk

ISBN 0 7499 2390 3

Text design by Paul Saunders
Edited by Louise Crathorne
Illustrations by Megan Hess

This book has been printed on paper manufactured
with respect for the environment using wood from
managed sustainable resources

Printed and bound in Great Britain by Bookmarque Ltd, Croydon, Surrey

Dedication

To James and William Ivens – the most wonderful
brothers and eligible bachelors in the world.

Contents

Acknowledgements

Thanks again to Alice Davis, Jana Sommerlad and all at Piatkus for their enthusiasm, Megan Hess for her illustrations and Ali Gunn at Curtis Brown for looking after me. Stefan – you are a prolific proofreader and I owe you big-time. Tina Weaver and Mel Brodie: thanks for not working me too hard at the day job (ha, ha!). Big shout going out to the girls in the know (Sarah Byne, Meredith Davies, Melissa Donnelly, Jacqueline Cohen, Catherine Harding, Jo Hewison, Claire Irvin, Lucy Nichols, Deirdre O'Brien, Kate Philpin, Karen Rollison, Claire Steele, Rose St Louis), and to the boys who should know better (Jonathan Clayton-Jones, Alan Greenhalgh, James Healy, Lee Holden) for their real- life research.

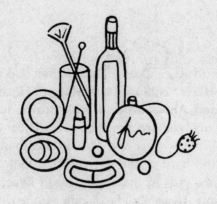

Introduction

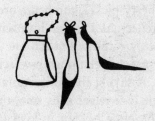

LOVE LIFTS US UP where we belong... Love is a many-splendoured thing... All you need is love... It's better to have loved and lost than never to have loved at all... and so on, and so on...

When it comes down to life's big question: 'Why are we here?' most people would answer: 'To be happy and self-fulfilled'. But even for a modern girl who's content doing her own thing, dating someone amazing can speed up this process. A good relationship can make you feel better than a pay rise, a decent holiday or a new pair of shoes. But who with? That's the tricky bit. And where can you find the one for you?

For the purposes of this book and your sanity, I'd like to propose that there is more than just the perfect 'one' somewhere out there. The available selection of worthwhile, long-term partners isn't as limited as all those slushy novels would have you believe. This isn't anti-romanticism, or naïve idealism, but a healthy dose of realistic mathematics. There are so many variables to consider that it would be foolish to approach the dating game without an awareness of them. Think about it. For example, not only does everyone have different sides to their personalities and feel attracted to hundreds of different-looking people, but also – and even worse – people all change as they get older. So my first tip is to stop panicking.

I had the first-kiss teenage fumbler, the sixth-form poet, the university cherry picker, the heart-breaking rogue, and the brooding intellectual. I was in love with them all – truly and wholeheartedly – and with each one I encountered different dating disasters, relationship-wreckers and make or break decisions. A saying that unfortunately is true is that the course of true love never runs smooth. But for all of us with a bit of fight left, all is fair in love and war, so get out there. Start pulling, charming, hypnotising and cruising. After all – you can smile with a mate, be nurtured by your family, and get praise from your colleagues – but there's nothing like a bloody good snog from someone you fancy to really make you feel fantastic.

Over the next ten chapters, I will aim to download every dating tip, hint, disaster and success that has ever entered my brain. That's not to say I'm some perfect dating queen – far from it, I've been dumped, two-timed, you name it – but with a bit of advice, from friends, family, experts and magazines, I got through the other side... and even managed to break a few hearts myself.

The one thing I promise is to help you learn more about yourself through your encounters with other people: Who makes you happy? What do you want to be doing at the weekend? Are you a mouse in bed or do you want to be having earth-shattering orgasms with a judo expert at the top of Everest? You shouldn't rule out any options until you've covered them all. If you've only thought you're worthy of a local guy who puts you down, think again.

Modern girls have everything at their fingertips – and don't the men just know it.

So good luck, get glammed up and go hell for leather on finding a man who makes you feel amazing... or failing that, a varied selection who help pass the time. Life's too short to take cold showers.

Chapter One

Love is a battlefield

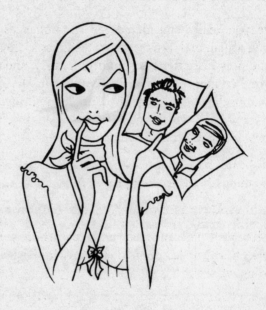

I N THE MOVIES, love is something that just happens to find you – at the supermarket, at work; Kate Winslet found it on a sinking ship for God's sake. And while in real life Leonardo DiCaprio isn't likely to ask you to go below decks, the beauty of it is that lasting love is out there for everyone – you just might have to work a bit harder, that's all. When love strikes, you have to know what to do with it. As the girl scouts say, be prepared. There's no point lusting after the man in the office if you stumble and splutter every time he approaches the photocopier. There's no point lingering outside McDonald's if every time the sexy burger-flipper approaches, you suffer from an involuntary bout of flatulence. No way, girl. Love is a battlefield and you need to get yourself armed.

No more lonely nights?

Have you really considered the consequences of all this getting-a-man malarkey? I know the grass is always greener, so you may lust after the stability, security, and regular sex of your committed sisters (committed in the relationship sense, not the mental), but there are many things that single girls get to do which must be considered before getting involved with another. So remember single girls get to:

◆ eat beans on toast every night of the week without a man moaning about needing proper food;

◆ fart in bed without ruining the feminine mystique;

◆ roll home drunk and puke in the bathroom without being seen, heard or lectured by a man who wishes he'd been doing what she has;

◆ spend their own money how they please;

◆ spend time with their own friends rather than having to be polite to partner's weird ones;

◆ forget about shaving until early May;

◆ be fab at their jobs without making a man feel inferior;

◆ run home to Mum when feeling ill;

◆ miss out on updates from his mum when he's feeling ill;

◆ book holidays to the Greek isles with the pure intention of having safe sex with some hunk on the beach;

◆ watch reruns of *Sex and The City* without feeling like they're letting the side down.

So that's settled then. Put the book down, being single rules. Or does it? Well in the short term maybe… but after a while the thrill of casual sex, drunkenly embarrassing yourself in public, coming over all Spice Girls *à la* 1996 with your girl-friends and eating microwave meals for one loses its (limited) appeal. You've got a heart, you think to yourself, maybe I should just use it.

Dating fatigue

So you've been dating for five, ten, fifteen years? Still single? Being out on the scene sounds glamorous and fun to those in long-term relationships, but in reality it can be tedious, tiring, expensive and bad for the liver. If you fancy a break, take one. Get off the scene and concentrate on yourself. Ignore your mother and her constant chat about becoming a grandmother. If you're despondent about dating, who'll have you? Take a chill pill and don't worry about missing out.

What is it that you really, really want?

If you do want to go on a manhunt, before you start prowling the streets of your local town, it's worth deciding what you want to get out of it. Nothing ever happens how you hope it will but you should at least set yourself a rough agenda. What are you looking for? Are you dating for fun, for the future, or for love? Are you worried about finding a man just because all your other friends have? Are you being pressured by your parents to settle down? Is the housing market in your area so extortionate the only way you can imagine getting a foot on the property ladder is by co-habiting? Are you worried you're an asexual/lesbian and this is your last bid to be 'normal'? Have you had an unworn wedding dress in your wardrobe for three years that's haunting you into marriage? Whatever your reason, who cares – we're living in a liberal society, just as long as you know what you're in for and arm yourself against emotional and physical hurt. Without sounding negative from the start, let's call this dating damage limitation.

Dating after disaster

We've already established the path of true love never did run smooth, so undoubtedly you will have been mucked up emotionally by relationships past. Whether you spent your teens moping after an older unrequited love, screwed over a parents' dream by snogging other men when you were at university, or had irreconcilable differences with your first husband, your love map is placed in front of you and you have to decide whether to regret the past, or get on with the future.

Love after love

Relationships don't come with a guidebook or a guarantee. People hope they have chosen the right person to spend time with but circumstances get difficult, life can throw strange things at you, and people's sensibilities change. As a resolutely single friend once said to me: 'I like Mars bars at the moment, but in five years' time I might not even fancy a nibble. I can't commit to one bar of chocolate for the rest of my life.' It's a cynical view perhaps but what I'm trying to say is that as long as you went into a relationship with honesty, love and hope, then you shouldn't be too hard on yourself if it has to come to an end and can look forward to falling in love again.

When can you start dating again?

Many of you may not want to date for a long time; in fact another man is the last thing you want. A serious split for modern girls is often a bolt for freedom – an attempt to reclaim their lifestyle, personality and youth before monotonous matrimony swallows it. However, once you've got through the various stages of failure, guilt, anger and loneliness, you may feel inclined to fall in love again.

How to get back on the single scene

Chances are things will have changed if you've been in a serious relationship for a long time – and I'm not talking about recognising the current dance anthem and the favoured cocktail of the moment. When you were first snapped up, many of your friends could have still been young, free and single alongside you. As time moves on, they're more likely to be older, buddied-up and taken. Hopefully you will have a few single mates remaining who are willing to accompany you on a manhunt. If all your friends are sensibly taken – and they aren't offering to fix you up with their love boat's mates – go and make new friends, or explore other groups who you haven't socialised with before. Go out after work with your colleagues, agree to go into town with your siblings' posses, or start attending social functions at your gym. You can't really start going out to bars and nightclubs alone unless they are specially organised singles nights. Your confidence may be shaky enough after a difficult divorce without having to walk into bars full of men on your own.

Finding a new partner

Unless splitting up was a mutual decision, one of you will be ready to date long before the other one. Even if you agree that you've grown apart and should separate, one person may still hanker after the past more than the other one. That is why both parties should enter the single scene discreetly and politely. They should not brag to mutual friends about their conquests or go to the favoured haunts of their ex-husband flaunting a new beau. It's going to hurt when you find out your ex has found a new soul mate. You may feel pain, regret and a plethora of could-have-beens. But life moves on and if you were made for each other, you'd still be together. Try to abstain from passing judgement and slagging off new dates. Concentrate on yourself. As long as there aren't children involved, you can date new people without worrying too much about how, what and when. When you do meet a new man, if he asks, tell the truth. You don't want to build a web of lies that you then have to retract as you get closer.

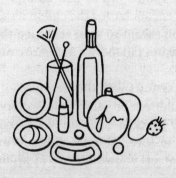

MEL, 40

❝Asking my first husband for a divorce was the most painful thing I ever had to do. I still loved him; I just wasn't in love with him anymore. I not only had to deal with my own regret and sadness but the guilt of being the one calling the shots. Although I couldn't date – or have sex – for a long time after separating, when I finally did meet someone special enough to be with, I still had lots of issues. I worried that my new partner would see me as a scarlet woman who broke hearts and promises. Luckily the new guy did trust me and we've now been married for ten years.❞

If you have children...

Children are always the first priority. My own parents got divorced when I was eight years old and I was unaware of my mother dating until I was introduced to the man she later married. Rather sensibly, my mother didn't want to introduce us to a string of men who might not stay in our lives. We had been traumatised enough. She did go out on dates – but she didn't stay overnight and we certainly didn't have to face any strangers over the breakfast table. The other extreme can be just as bad though – abstaining from any romantic encounter for the children's sake is not a good move, you don't want to start resenting them. One day the kids will grow up, fall in love and move out.

When it gets serious with the new guy

Your ex should not be informed of every Tom, Dick and Harry you've shacked up with since your split but once you've fallen in love, it's only polite to inform him. Likewise, if he contacts you with news of his imminent move-in or wedding, try to act with grace and goodwill and don't demand an invite.

The grass is always greener

When you get back on the single scene after being in a steady relationship, you're going to go through a phase of regretting your choice (if you were the 'chucker') or falling further into the depths of depression (if you were the 'chucked'). Don't panic and think things will stay this way forever. You're bound to look at your last relationship through rose-tinted glasses when you are faced with a gaggle of unwholesome, unattached men. Suddenly, you'll forget about the arguments, the bossiness, and the untidiness and only recall the closeness. But staying in an unhealthy relationship is for the lazy, modern girl – not the fulfilled, modern girl. Don't go back to the future.

Preparing the groundwork

1. Firstly it's time for bluntness – no one is going to want you if you're a mess – on the outside or inside. A relationship will only work if you're offering something more than desperation, self-doubt or blind panic.

2. Your wardrobe must also be up to the challenge. It's pretty sub-standard to wear the same outfit on the first few dates so you need to have a few options at the ready, i.e. no kebab stains, or see-through (overly suggestive) skirts. Also check your underwear – more on this in Chapter 5.

3. Your bank account could take a bit of a battering, so save money on household appliances, travel, birthday presents

for your friends (they'll forgive you) and spend it all on drinks for Dutch courage, gym membership, and that sexy top that makes your boobs look fab. But seriously, more and more men like a modern girl who will hold her own and is therefore in control – unless of course you plan on snogging (and snagging) a millionaire. More on that later too.

4. Your health should be at optimum level. Successful sharking, and then hopefully dating, involves heavy drinking, late nights and lots of stress. Will he, won't he? Should I swing from the chandelier in that flameproof negligee on our first date? All of the above take it out on the immune system so start knocking back those vitamins now, before you get knocked out. Try investing in some of those 'busy woman' formulas you see in the chemist – not only do they help, but they'll also make you feel very important as you march up the aisle to make your purchase.

5. It is important that you have space in your life for any relationship that might begin. Now may not be the time to start that evening class or adopt a Chinese baby. It will be vital to make your new partner feel like they're the centre of your world at least until you've got him hooked.

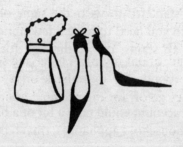

NB Tread carefully in the early stages. Don't make the fatal flaw of abandoning your circle of die-hard friends as soon as Mr Maybe-Right says: 'Are you free next Thursday?' As soon as Mr Maybe-Right says: 'I think we want different things' – you'll need them more than ever. That is if they haven't deleted your email address and burnt you in effigy, which they'd have every right to do. A modern girl never abandons her friends. A relationship will change things so tread carefully in the early stages.

6. Be careful not to lose the plot completely over the prospect of new love. If you're lucky enough you might have a sympathetic boss who will overlook a few misty-eyed daydreams out of the window and lots of flushed giggling on the work phone. If you're not, then concentrate, girl – you can't afford to throw away your professional and personal reputation. My boss recently referred to working for our magazine as the best contraceptive in London – we're too busy to even think about sex, let alone actually have it.

7. Ask your family to keep their noses out – there's no better passion killer than a mother who wants to find what your new date is like in bed. I never went off a man so quickly as when my auntie, trying to find out if I'd lost my virginity to my university bloke, suggested we 'run down a few ways to make love without having sex'. Puke. I don't want to think about my parents having sex, let alone the other way round. Try to embark on a flamboyant love affair as they go off for their annual holiday.

Finding a partner in crime

Single friends are also useful for a number of reasons:

- They make you feel normal.

- They don't care about garden furniture either so you can have a conversation about important things. Like whether the sexy new guy in your office is gay or just well groomed.

- They are available on Friday nights.

- They accept that four hours to get ready is a reasonable amount of time.

- They don't agree with your 'taken' friends that night-clubs are dirty, overpriced and full of losers, in fact, they think the music is great and the cocktails are even better.

NB Always remember you are in competition. Unless your idea of a perfect man is a blond midget from Michigan while your friend solely goes for 7 ft Eskimos, you're bound to overlap on the 'I fancy him' chart a few times. This causes resentment, fear and often strip-to-the-waist-and-fight-me-bitch squabbling. So if hunting with a pack of fellow up-for-it girls do lay the groundwork first.

Sharking rules

As per ancient customs, above all else, the rule to be observed when playing the game of love is: 'I saw him first so he's mine. I don't care if he's your type, or if he's offered to buy you a drink. I said I liked him while you were still flirting with Roger from accounts. So there.' All friends who wish to remain friends while trying to find a date should strictly follow this guideline:

> **NB Only go out on the prowl with girls you know you can trust.** There is a girl in my wider friendship circle who cannot even be left in the same football stadium as someone else's prospective date. It seems some girls need the reassurance of a man's attractiveness from their friends, only feeling compelled to make a move once that man is already earmarked.

Been there, done that

No matter how needy you get (I won't say desperate – that's so not the look for a modern girl), try not to date a friend's ex. It may seem like a good idea at the time – after all you know where they've been (making out in your mate's car, for God's sake, yuk!) and who they've been with, which in today's sexually aware society might appear to be a good thing. Apart from the fact that it's not. It's bad enough having dodgy ex-girlfriends to deal with when you meet a new man. But imagine not being able to slag off said ex because she's your mate. As a loyal friend you'd never be able to enquire if her bum's bigger than yours, if she was quieter in bed or even if she put the chic into psychotic.

Better the devil you know?

While we're on the subject of exes, maybe we should quickly refer to your own. Winter's drawing in, perhaps Valentine's is only a few days away, perhaps all your girls have booked their summer holiday and you fancy a romantic trip to the Indian Ocean. Don't do it. Don't call the ex who you know still carries a flame for you because he tells your mates when he's pissed and has been known to leave pleading messages on your machine at midnight. Some people say better the devil you know, I'd argue familiarity breeds contempt. It's nice to believe in new beginnings and fresh starts, but baggage is baggage. Even if you reunite five years later, and he says he's forgotten all about that fling you had, it's not so simple. The first time things get spicy, all of your past sins could be brought back to haunt you. And can you truly forgive his gambling, bossiness and devotion to his mother in your new spirit of togetherness? In general, the argument against dating an ex is like premenstrual thighs, it holds a lot of water. I'm not saying reunion never works, but why not use a willing ex instead to improve your self-confidence, to know that men still find you attractive? Then take the time to work out from past relationships what has and hasn't worked for you, and go out and find yourself a baggage-less date.

Commencing battle

Once you've established what you're looking for, what you're trying to avoid and what the ideal outcome is you're ready to get going – so long as you've shaved your legs of course.

The desirable dater's emergency pack

All gorgeous girls who are ready to bestow some big love on a worthy man should keep the following in their handbag, or desk drawer:

- Bronzing powder to give you a healthy glow even after a busy day, hangover, or bout of food poisoning.

- Tights to look groomed after a fight with a revolving door or a spiky bush.

- Condoms – where and how you do it is your own business – just be safe.

- Clean pair of knickers in case you can't make it home.

- Mouth freshener, or chewing gum to be fresh the whole day through.

- Deodorant.

- Mobile phone – to inform your date of your late arrival and likewise your mother.

- Diary – to plan the next date while showing him how popular you are.

- A wallet full of cash – don't rely on him to pay, especially if you don't want to take it further. Just make sure you've got enough cash for a round of drinks and the cab ride home.

Oh no! Eau de desperado!

However keen you are to get your mitts on an eligible bachelor, don't act desperate. Men can smell it a mile off. Think about it from their point of view. Men think (we know the truth of course) that all women want is a husband, a gaggle of screaming kids, a dog, a rabbit and a country pile. This scares them witless. They think we're after their hearts, their money and their sperm – in that order. The more needy you appear in those first few conversations, the more he'll feel the need to back off. Try and see it their way: If a bloke you quite fancied asked what you'd call your first-born over the first bottle of Chablis, you'd back off a bit too.

When to go on the hunt?

Werewolves rely on the moon. Women rely on their mood. We all know that a certain time of the month is a washout as far as emotional stability is concerned. Those hormones will be racing so fast through your veins that you won't be able to keep hold of a mate, let alone a date. It's a stereotype but the week before menstruation, women are moody, stroppy, weepy, irrational and bloated. Then they bleed and get tummy ache. Then the only good phase of the whole cycle occurs – heightened sex drive. But because God is obviously a man, for horniest phase also read spottiest phase when no man would come near you.

So perhaps start your prowling when feeling at your emotional and physical peak – normally the week after your period. Pick a time when work is relatively stress-free (is there such a thing?) so you can devote more time to polishing your nails than paperwork. If you're looking to date by season, the most popular time is spring. The world is full of fresh hope, people have been going to the gym since January and the sun is at last shining. Although of course summer holidays are a good time to pull and Christmas makes everyone feel sentimental.

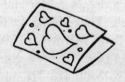

Playing the game

Try this quick quiz to find out if you're ready to play the game:

The game of love is like:
A. Chess – you check out lots of mates
B. Poker – you don't open up until you know he's the one
C. Monopoly – you stake your claim straightaway

When you like a man you say to your friends:
A. He's hot – but there are still plenty more fish in the sea
B. He's nice, we're taking it easy
C. I like his surname – I think I'll take it if we marry

The morning after first-time sex you're:
A. Back home with your own beauty products
B. Enjoying a quick cup of coffee with him before making an exit
C. Planning a day trip with him to the countryside

Mostly As
You know how to play the field – but perhaps you're a little too cynical and well dated. Try to enjoy the romance and keep focused on one fella, rather than a whole gaggle of them. You won't miss out if you commit, you know. And you won't get your heart broken every time.

Mostly Bs
You want to find the one and you don't mind waiting for him. You genuinely like men and enjoy their company but you don't go all silly over the first one to pay you a compliment. Well done you. You've got it sussed. You do protect yourself but you have to when you're playing such serious games.

Mostly Cs

You don't want to admit you're dating... you're looking for a husband. Sorry honey, you've got to lighten up. Men will get a whiff of you and run. You're sweet, kind and finished with all this immature game-playing, but try not to lay all your cards out at once. You'll get trampled on.

Secrets of Success...

♦ Be yourself. There's no point putting on a show to snare a man if you remove the mask as soon as you move in together. If you're not comfortable with yourself, no one else will be. (You can use artistic licence to exaggerate your good points if necessary.)

♦ Learn from your mistakes. If you have a catalogue of disasters, try to see any common patterns of unsuitability.

♦ However, don't spend too long analysing the past. It's called the past for a reason.

♦ Beware of the rebound. Modern girls are big enough and beautiful enough to look after themselves, but when hearts get broken, even the most sensible of girls can try and heal them too quickly. There's no rush. There's no shame in being on your own. And there's no shame in falling for the wrong guy in a bid to escape an unhappy marriage. Anything that gets you away from a life of misery is a good thing. Just don't marry your rebound, give him your divorce settlement cash or have his baby straight out of the starting blocks.

♦ Don't assume that because you didn't get hitched, it wasn't as serious or as hard to get over. If you live together, you will still have to sort out the lease on your rented flat or terminate the mortgage. If you have children, splitting up will be trickier than if you were married because the law doesn't state exactly what you can and can't have. In some cases you should consider hiring an independent financial adviser or lawyer to help you decide who should get what. Give yourself time and ignore helpful relatives who say: 'Well at least you didn't marry him!'

◆ Don't expect sympathy from any of your ex-husband's family or friends, even if they admit they couldn't live with him themselves. They're being loyal, which is good. You'd expect your friends and family to do the same.

◆ If you're separated but still living under the same roof, don't bring back new dates. That's cruel and unnecessary – pack an overnight bag and stay at his.

◆ Never suggest double-dating with your ex-husband. Even if you are still friends, the combination of booze and flirting is asking for trouble.

◆ Don't get into slagging off your ex to new partners – you'll only look as though you still care a little too much and they worry about what they're getting into.

◆ In a bid to establish domestic bliss, don't rush into cashing in your divorce settlement and settling into a new mortgage with the new man. Chill out and live on your own for a bit.

◆ Divorce will make you feel sad, empty, lonely, guilty and stupid. That's taken for granted. It should also make you feel like you've got a second chance at finding your soul mate. Learn from your mistakes. Don't push your past relationships to the back of your mind. Remember what made you happy, what made you sad, and try and work out your own behavioural problems to stop the same mistakes happening again.

♦ Don't think that men will judge you for being married before. There is something ultimately sexy about dating a divorcee... think Marilyn Monroe and Elizabeth Taylor.

♦ When looking for a new partner, do not simply try to replace the conveniences of having a man around the house. You're looking for love, not a second-hand gardener, taxi driver, or accountant.

♦ Unless you've always been tempted to try a bit of ladylove action, do not go down the lesbian route. Sometimes it's tempting to joke that men are all useless heartbreakers and women would be better off without them... which, when we're acting rationally, we know isn't strictly true. When you finally get over the painful split you may be embarrassed about the lipstick lesbo routine you tried on with the bisexual flirt from the office.

♦ If you're new to the dating game – don't confuse sex with love.

♦ Avoid crash dieting and comfort bingeing – you won't be healthy enough to rejoin the dating game.

♦ You can't hurry love. Enough said.

♦ Remember – if you're happy, those around you will be happy for you. The road to happiness may be difficult to follow, but your real friends will travel with you over any rocky terrain. There's a bit of American psycho-babble for you... Geri Halliwell eat your heart out.

♦ Work out if you're looking for a few fun dates or a serious relationship and don't get confused with what the man you've met is offering. You can't make someone love you if they don't. Don't build up a date into a life-long love affair.

◆ Try to make the most of being single – it will make settling down a lot easier and perversely make you look a more attractive relationship option.

◆ Get your friends' advice on what kind of guy suits you and where you could find him. They know you better than anyone – even, dare I say it, your parents when it comes to who you fancy, your attitude to love etc. But don't take anyone's advice as gospel. Everyone has issues and their own agenda.

◆ Don't openly state you're on a mission to meet a man. Your mum will start planning her wedding outfit, your friends will ask for a progress report every time they see you, and you could end up feeling like a failure if you don't succeed within a certain amount of time.

◆ Be confident. You are fan-bloody-tastic. Remember that during the trials and tribulations, ups and downs of the next few weeks, months or even years.

◆ And if all else fails... don't get too depressed about being single – people in relationships are on average 2.5 kg heavier than their single sisters.

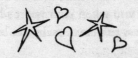

Chapter Two

Looking for love: Friends

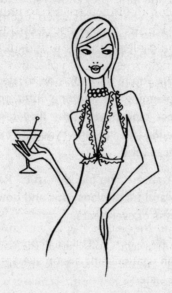

FRIENDS ARE GREAT, aren't they? They warm your heart on cold winter mornings, look after you when you're sick, console you when your heart's been broken... and hopefully have access to many an eligible bachelor who is just perfect for you.

Friendly fixers

If the reason you want a man is because of the shelf-sitting syndrome (an illness affecting women worried they'll be left on the shelf for the rest of their life), then ask your friends for their tips or recommendations. Unless you absolutely hate their partners, i.e. you suspect your best friend has no taste in men because her boyfriend Dave is an idiot, and would rather live life alone than meet a Dave clone, coupled-up mates are the best sources of fresh, young blood. Not only are they not interested for themselves, but also they are keen for all of their friends to join their LUNB club (we're **L**oved **U**p, we're **N**ot being **B**oring honest guv club). Nothing would please them more than turning their funky, free, fun single friends (i.e. you) into stay-at-home girlfriends who refuse invites to Westlife after-shows to sit in with a pizza and a good video. The less single girls out there, the more comfortable they feel with their own choices. It's Bridget Jones's Smug Marrieds gone berserk... But these couples aren't smug, they're fearful. Fearful of that other life they lived way, way back. Take advantage of your friends' fears and ask them to either dish up some dishy guys, or accompany you on the pilgrimage to local bars so you can find for yourself what her and Dave have. She'll love the vindication. You'll love the fact you won't find them swapping phone numbers in the toilets with the cute barman you had your eyes on. Everyone's a winner.

Making a move on your mate's mate

This is difficult territory. Unless your friend has specifically tried to fix you up with someone, it probably means she thinks you are an unlikely couple. Look at it from her point of view. Fixing up friends with friends has a lot of pros and cons...

Pros

She'll get to play cupid and see two friends happy. They will love her and buy her lots of drinks in the pub. She has a good chance of being godmother to their firstborn because, after all, without her, there wouldn't be a baby to christen.

Cons

Her two friends will fall madly in love and not have time to talk to her anymore. She will be left out of the loop until they split up, when she will be called upon to pick sides and then rearrange her social calendar so the two never bump into each other again. Or, she may allow her friends to start dating, only to realise that she herself has feelings for him and now she either has to act like a stroppy bitch or have her heart broken.

So before you delve into a friend's address book for Mr Right, make sure she's not harbouring any flames of passion for him or hidden fears that you'll be really bad for each other.

NB Dating a friend's sibling is almost always a no-no. If people get jealous when their mates pair up and get close, imagine what it's like if suddenly you know more about your friend's brother than she does. She loves you in the right context (as a shoulder to cry on, dance partner or holiday companion) but she won't be keen for you to overstep the mark. Opening presents with you on Christmas morning while her parents fawn over you may be a little too much for your friendship to take. If you and a friend's sibling do get close, try to imagine how she feels and don't become part of the family too soon.

Blind dates

Why, oh why do we agree to them? Because we trust our friends, that's why. We have similar taste in clothes and music, so we must have similar taste in men. Think again. Before you give your mate free rein to fix you up with the bloke from the pub that she would be dating if she wasn't already hitched, do the taste test. Compare and contrast a variety of men (make sure you cover the extremes, i.e. throw in a few Salman Rushdies, Jamie Olivers and Elton Johns amongst the Brad Pitts and George Clooneys) and if you have similar results, trust her. Give general guidelines as to required height, girth, weight, age etc.

SARAH, 27

❝ Remember your friend's idea of 'good-looking and great personality' is not always the same as yours. I went on a blind date when I was about 18; a colleague thought her husband's friend and I would get on really well and I agreed to meet him. Sensibly we had our blind date in a restaurant I was working in at the time so I knew people. Well, her description of tall, dark and handsome definitely wasn't the same as mine. His hair was like Dracula's: it came to a point in the middle of his forehead and looked as if he had poured a bottle of cooking oil over it. His leather jacket with shoulder pads and brown suede shoes were really off-putting. I immediately knew I didn't fancy this guy but as the girl who set us up was present to introduce us I couldn't pretend I wasn't there. The conversation was fine, although we didn't have much in common, but I managed about one and a half hours with several long toilet breaks. I had arranged for a friend to call me halfway through the evening as my get-out clause. I employed the excuse of a distraught friend who had just had a major row with her partner and left the blind date without even bothering to take the guy's phone number. Harsh but fair, I didn't want to get his hopes up. ❞

NB Don't tell your friend off if the blind date is a disaster.
Unless she is particularly cruel, she had your best interests
at heart. Maybe suggest next time that you meet any likely
lads at a wider social event – like a dinner party or cocktail
reception.

Weak in the presence of beauty

Of course blind dates can also leave you face-to-face with
perfection. And you're not prepared. And you feel a bit
silly. If he doesn't do a runner, stick with it. He might not be
as looks-obsessed as you... and most women are more
attractive than they admit anyway.

CLAIRE, 28

  ❝ I had a blind date with what turned out to be an absurdly
attractive guy. We are talking stunning and my friend didn't
think to warn me. She must have been madly in love with
her own boyfriend because she passed him on to me. He
was so perfect that I lost the power of speech and could only
say yes or no. He tried to make polite conversation, asked
me about my life, my career, and my family. I said
'mmmmm, yeaahhhh' or 'oohhhh naahhhh'. He soon left
me at the bar to die slowly of regret. So too much of a good
thing does exist. ❞

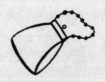

Five top tips for escaping bad blind dates

1. A pre-planned phone call, or text message halfway through the evening from a trusted friend.

2. Suddenly develop a nasty cough, say you are going to vomit, that you have a headache, or similar.

3. If he's really not your type but isn't taking your polite hints, start flirting with the waiter, barman, or cloakroom attendant and openly ask for their number.

4. Start crying and say you haven't got over your old love and/or he's just appeared over the other side of the restaurant and it really would be a good idea for him to leave before he gets beaten up.

5. Don't drink. Drive yourself to the blind date so that you are able to make a quick getaway in your car. Sometimes you don't have to make any excuses – you're never going to meet the guy again. Remember – these are tips for escaping bad blind dates, I'm not advocating doing this if the guy has offended you by not liking Ricky Martin.

> **NB Get a second opinion.** Another friend arranged to have a best mate and her husband already positioned in the meeting place. They were under strict instructions not to acknowledge her. Then, when she arrived with her blind date, not only did she have a reassuring back-up but, as a result of their anonymous presence, she was able to have someone to discuss her pros and cons with the next day.

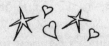

Attending other people's work dos

This sounds awful doesn't it? It's bad enough going to your own drink-fuelled, sweaty-manager-laden, office-gossip fest twice yearly... but attending a corporate function where you don't know anyone from Adam sounds hellish (unless of course Adam just happens to be a 6 ft 3 hunk of steel with a warm tan and a degree in economics). Look at it this way: attending an office function with your mate is a clever way of cutting through crap. She knows his job title, his social habits, and his prospects and maybe – if she works in the personnel department – his salary and pension plan details (all highly confidential of course but she can drop you a few hints). He's bound to have drunkenly snogged another girl in the office so you can even get a tongue-action low-down.

Although you have primarily accepted the invite to go sharking, remember your friend's reputation is at stake. Obviously she chose to invite you out of all the other modern girls she knows because you're fun, sociable and intelligent – so act it. Don't get drunk and initiate a canapé-throwing contest, she'll never invite you to a work function again. Don't overcompensate for the invite and offer to give her boss a blow-job in the toilets (unless he's single, sexy and you think he might repay the compliment). This will definitely get around the office and your mate will be labelled 'whore's friend' by the following Monday. Don't wear anything too over the top and don't spill red wine on the managing director's wife' silk chemise. Got it? Sorted. Observing those rules you can ask your friend to point you in the direction of her highest paid, or best-looking, colleagues... you might as well start at the top and not go straight to the accountancy rejects. When you get chatting, your friend should subtly disappear to the bar, or toilets, to let you see if you can maintain the banter on your own. To keep it casual, ask about the office characters, the boss's temper, and your friend's professional disasters. Act impressed. Make his job sound interesting even if you're convinced he's a sucker for working in a paper factory. If you like him, great. You don't have to push anything. Your friend is bound to bump into him within a few days. She can get the low-down, start sending out a few joke emails to both of you and suggest a night at the pub over the road from the office. You can show up fashionably late after attending another wonderful party and make a beeline for him.

Your friend will like having a mate date a colleague for a while. It makes socialising with the two groups a heck of a lot easier, and she'll get kudos in the office for having fit and up-for-it mates. The boss will also see her as sociable and a good matchmaker and may invite her to more out-of-office events. However, if you get too close too quickly, don't leave her out. In her eyes she owns a bit of the relationship – so debrief her on any large manoeuvres before she hears that you've moved in together on the office grapevine. Similarly, don't commiserate with her on not getting the pay rise, promotion, or new office if she doesn't mention it first. She may not know yet or may have wanted to tell you herself. This kind of problem occurs when friends fix you up with any of their social circle so beware.

Dinner dates

The oldest dating trick in the book seems to be to invite single friends together and force them to sit next to each other while eating spaghetti. Friends who don't mind slaving away over a hot stove and cleaning their house in order for you to get laid are friends indeed. Dinner parties are notoriously gruelling to prepare for, so the fact that you're a singleton must be a real issue for her. Whether she is happily paired off and wants the same for all her mates or whether she just likes being the hostess with the mostest, who cares! Enjoy her hospitality – single girls don't get many opportunities to get their five servings of fresh fruit and vegetables every day. And meeting men in the comfort of your friend's home rather than in a packed bar can be liberating. You don't have to worry about making contact, and then if it goes well, you don't have to worry about closing hours – you can comfortably drink into the small hours when a local cab firm will take you home.

Party for two?

It's obvious why you two singletons have been placed amongst three couples for dinner. The other couples are there to show you how wonderful being in a couple is, and you two are there to be fixed up. If you know from the start you're not interested, offer to help your mate in the kitchen and inform her so. It doesn't mean you get to go home, but it might stop her and her partner from making suggestive comments. You can then adopt a friendly, jovial tone with your dinner date – that won't be misconstrued as flirting. For example, refer to film stars you fancy but don't keep going on about the guy in the gym that you're obsessed with. Chances are you've met before if briefly so conversation should be okay – you'll have mutual friends staring at you intently with their beady eyes after all. If you do like the guy, joke about being fixed up so he knows you know this is kind of a love thing and that you're relaxed about it. Make sure you're sitting next to him at dinner but make sure you talk to the rest of the group too, otherwise you'll come across as unsociable and clingy.

Double-dating

This seems safe, but also a bit sad. How can you really get to know someone while your friend is kicking you under the table and encouraging you to join her on the dance floor? Also, make sure your friend isn't setting you up with the dud mate of her date. In her desperation to get Prince Charming out for the night, she might have promised his ugly chum a snog with her fab friend. It's flattering that she feels you're attractive bait – and we must help friends wherever possible in their bid to find true love – but don't feel bad if it's just not your thing.

However, it's important to set the rules before a joint dating mission:

◆ If you and your mate are out together and spot two likely lads, decide which one you are each going for early on. You don't want to both be fighting over the one with the Porsche after a few hours. Hair-pulling is so unattractive in the over-fives.

◆ Make sure you both have your cab fare home and a mobile phone in case one of the set-ups is more successful than the other.

◆ Don't tell lots of in-jokes or bore the fellas with stories of your schooldays etc. Until a man is in love with you, he doesn't care if you got sent out of Miss Pilkington's geography lesson for farting.

◆ Don't encourage each other to drink too much. It's not a girls' night out – you're trying to look alluring, which is difficult to do with tequila breath and vomit in your hair.

◆ Don't introduce the boys to your private world of line dancing, or your high-speed grapevine to *99 Red Balloons;* you may find it amusing but it may scare anyone else.

◆ Try to talk to your friend's date as well as your own. This will make you look sociable and intelligent when they compare notes later and you may also uncover some useful info to tell your mate in the cab on the way home.

◆ Agree to sell each other – don't tell embarrassing stories or discuss disastrous past relationships.

◆ Don't go to the loos together. Not only is it infantile but also your dates will get suspicious.

◆ Be different. If you drink, eat, think and dance the same, you may appear more like the Beverley Sisters than the hot, young things you really are.

◆ If the double date goes well, suggest going out separately next time. Sure, do the foursome thing in a few dates' time but try not to settle into the comfort of joint dates. You won't really get to know each other properly in company.

Hitching a ride

It's widely known that many couples have got together at their friends' weddings. You know the score, there's romance in the air, everyone's up for a good time, and you look great. What could be better? You grew up with the bride; he works with the groom – whatever – wedding days are perfect matchmaking occasions.

Five hints for meeting a man at a friend's wedding

1. Play down your eagerness to catch the bouquet. You don't want to look too desperate. Instead enthusiastically applaud the lucky girl.

2. Check the table plan beforehand; if you've got a cute guy's name, you may be able to do some hasty rearranging. Don't go too far with this – it's your friend's day after all.

3. If you get close to the guy of your dreams, position yourself near the elderly relatives in attendance. It's likely they'll start cooing over how beautiful the pair of you are together etc.

4. Book a room at the reception venue; you don't want to be forced into rushing off just as the evening is getting interesting.

5. Have fun and be sociable. Being a modern girl who holds her own will ensure she gets maximum attention from all the eligible bachelors still under the romantic influence of the happy couple.

Foreign affair

If your friends aren't much use at home, take them away. Twist their arm to travel with you to find a date. I'm not talking about just going away and praying each night for a holiday romance – I'm talking about actually getting on a plane with only one thing on your mind. Meeting a man. Sod the tan (I know, I know, hard for us girls to do) and go to some more unusual places specifically set up to cater for the single and proactive. It's best to take a friend so you have the confidence to go into bars and restaurants – and you have an escape route from any creepy guys (which there will be plenty of).

NB Holidaying with a friend as a single girl is all about balance. You don't want to abandon your mate as soon as you meet the señor or monsieur of your dreams. If she hasn't been as lucky, make sure you include her in your arrangements as much as possible. Make time to do things together like you planned to. Think about it, if the situation were reversed – you wouldn't appreciate being abandoned in some foreign clime with only the hotel staff for company whilst your friend is whisked off to meet her new Greek family in the neighbouring villages.

Dating your own friends

Is dating your own friends a good idea? This is a difficult question, and one that every single girl with an array of lovely male friends has asked herself at some point. We've all seen *When Harry Met Sally*. You're in on your own on a Friday night, your old mate from school Johnny Available calls and ask if he should come over with a takeaway and a video. You say yes. You don't bother to put any make-up on or brush your teeth because he loves you just the way you are. He arrives, you have a laugh, being on your own doesn't seem so bad... and then, after he's gone, you think to yourself: 'If only I fancied him.'

Try not to confuse extreme friendliness and compatibility with the full-on love thing. In a moment of weakness, you may believe that sexual attraction is overrated and that you're better off with a confidante who cares, a bit like Boy George and his famous preference for cups of tea over sex.

If you think you have a more than platonic soft spot for a buddy, go out on your own for the night and get lashed. Doctors wouldn't advise it but sometimes alcohol acts like truth juice. Get him tipsy and make a drunken pass. If it feels good and he doesn't bite your head off with: 'Get away from me you drunken tart,' maybe you could be more than just good friends.

Prepare yourself for a full-on love affair straight away – you can't shirk about playing games because you both already know far too much about each other. You don't have to go through the formalities of first dates, meeting friends and family etc. Dating mates can be great – you have common ground and more than just a sexual chemistry, you actually like each other! Just don't rush into things assuming that a friend will make a good lover... if you were destined to be together you might have realised it sooner, not when you were feeling a bit low.

REBECCA, 33

⁶ After spending far too much time getting my hopes dashed and my heart broken, I decided to look a little closer to home. My story is embarrassingly chick-lit. The boy in the background who I would turn to when my love life went sour *became* my love life. I'd always assumed that because James and I started out as mates – and there wasn't the initial 'let's shag' thing going on – that we were destined to be just friends. Not true. We did move things on a little too quickly because he couldn't try any of his old tricks on me and we knew each other's quirks. ⁹

Passing the time with a shag-chum

Rather than pretending to be madly in love with one of your mates, why not set up a system where you can use each other for regular sex? If you're single, healthy and happy to use each other as human sex toys (and risk developing stronger, unrequited feelings), this could be the answer to untold frustrations and unhappy one-night stands with strangers. Certain rules apply: some people won't approve of your informal shagathons so keep it quiet – *both* of you. When one or both of you start a new relationship, take a back seat without making a scene. Stay friends – that's what you are essentially anyway. And never, ever, ever tell new beaus about this relationship – jealousy is hard to handle and he may not understand how you can dislocate sex from love – it can seem rather cold. This really is one for the modern girls alone.

Secrets of Success

♦ Some people just don't fix up friends with friends full stop. And who can blame them – it's a dangerous game with lots of toxic waste if it goes wrong. Don't push it, unless you think your mate's next-door neighbour could be your soul mate.

♦ Never rub your friend's face in your new relationship. Imagine how you'd feel. She's been friends with Freddie Fixed-up for ten years and after two months you're now arguing with her over his favourite sandwich filling. Even if she's completely wrong, let it go.

♦ Don't listen to all she has to say. Although she might be happy for her friends to be getting together, she may resent being ousted from her prime position on his speed dial. Take information like 'his mother's a witch who hates career girls' with a pinch of salt. Your friend may subconsciously make things a little difficult for you.

♦ Ask your friend to dig through her photo albums for a photograph of your date – blind dates don't literally have to be 'blind'. An out-of-date picture is better than nothing. If there's no visual evidence of his suitability – get a second opinion if possible. Ask your friend's partner for a description.

♦ Don't date your parents' friends, and even be wary of dating the children of your parents' friends. Your mother and her cronies from the Bridge club may enjoy discussing your relationship, but you'll be expected to attend far too many social functions together to please the old folk. However, if parents' friends' son is a male supermodel, ignore the above. At least for a few weeks.

♦ Friends may be happy to fix you up at their expense at first, but you can't continue to use them as a dating service. If you click with one of their mates at a dinner party, get his number, and do your own thing next time. Their house is not a brothel. Sure, ask them to introduce you to a few eligible men but draw the line at sucking them dry of every available man in their address book. If it doesn't work after three fix-ups, accept that you may have to do the dating thing on your own.

◆ Spare your friends the details of your sex life. It's bad enough that they may have to watch two mates snogging; they don't need to know you've just installed a gimp room in the basement.

◆ If things don't work out, don't demand your friend takes sides. It will be difficult to know they still go out but it's not your place to demand s/he says goodbye because you have.

◆ Try not to make your friend piggy in the middle. It's accept-able in the first few weeks to call for feedback but after three dates you have to realise your love life isn't your friend's main concern. Her love life is. Give it a rest. If she has any stellar info, she'll volunteer it.

◆ Think twice about dating an ex-boyfriend-now-friend of a friend. It can be embarrassing enough stripping off in front of a man for the first time anyway, without thinking he's comparing your boobs with your mate's.

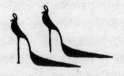

Chapter Three

Looking for love:
The professionals

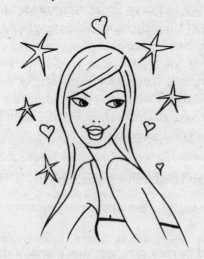

I F ONLY LOVE WAS LIKE light, we'd be able to find it every-where. Draw back the curtains in the morning and Mr Perfect is outside the window. Whoosh. Flick a switch and the man of your dreams enters the room. Unfortu-nately, people have to work a little harder than that and with modern life getting more and more stressful, solitary and selfish, finding someone worth dating might seem like an impossibility. But hang on, if we can put a man on the moon, and sausages in beans, we can get you a love interest. And the options are endless so chill out. There are an esti-mated eight million single adults in Britain alone. Time for a bit of marketing...

Advertising yourself

GSOH, and all that malarkey, has made placing a personal ad a bit of a joke. They seem to be associated with gay men, dwarf fetishists and married ladies looking for a bit of extra-curricular action. Yet as we get busier and women have to start looking for love in new places, advertising can be quick, cheap and easy. Some nationwide and most local newspapers have 'lonely heart' sections placed discreetly at the back, and many specialist magazines have sections for people looking for a particular type of person, be it gay, straight, swinging, sadomasochistic, fat, or over-50. Most of these publications will act as the middleman – and gather responses for you and pass them on to you in bulk (hoping that you get a good response).

Dos and Don'ts of selling yourself

◆ Do tell the truth… but not if you are an ex-convict with halitosis.

◆ Do be brief in your message; don't write a dissertation (it will cost you a fortune and you'll sound like you're over-compensating).

◆ Do sound keen. Don't sound desperate.

◆ Do use a reputable publication but don't print your home address or phone number.

◆ Do use a fake name if you feel uncomfortable but don't rechristen yourself Ms Whiplash… unless that's what you're after.

◆ Do say exactly what you're looking for in a guy, unless you're just after a millionaire.

◆ **Do** think carefully about who you tell about placing the ad. You don't want them judging you and any relationships that come from it.

◆ **Do** try more than once and **don't** get disheartened if the first batch of replies is abysmal... it could have been a slow week in love land.

KAREN, 44

❝ I had got bored with meeting blokes in pubs and night clubs, so one tipsy evening I sat down to advertise for a man in the local paper. In the first week I had 24 replies, so the task of sorting through them took a long time... although several went straight in the bin because they were from perverts! I whittled it down to one and I plucked up the courage to call him. We chatted for ages and he made me laugh a few times, so we made a date. It was raining and I had got to the pub car park early, so I watched as he parked his car and sat there not looking around to see if I was coming. I scuttled across the car park and tapped on his window. The poor thing was more nervous than I was but we had a good evening and time flew. He even admitted he was worried I'd had a bladder problem when I confessed all those trips to the loo were really telephone check-ins with my friend. We're now married so the ad worked. ❞

Secret agencies

A possibly more successful – if expensive – way of advertising yourself is to sign up to a dating agency. Going to a good – and by good I mean recommended, reputable and reasonable – agency is like finding a dating personal trainer... perfect for the stressed-out modern girl. Hand over cash, talk about yourself and then tell them what you want/need and give them an insight into your availability for dates. In theory, as soon as you've helped the experts make your web page or video, that's it. You're free to go and run the investment bank, edit a national newspaper or run 20 miles before breakfast, and let them take the strain of getting you a man. And in theory, they should be getting you the right one. Make no bones about what you need. If you live in London and they can only find you men from Inverness, you are within your rights to demand your money back and move on to another agency.

> **NB You are bloody fantastic.** Any modern man out there will be lucky if the dating agency suggest you as a possible match. Don't sell yourself short in the misguided belief that you're going to have to settle for something less than your normal expectation. Men exaggerate their positive attributes far more than women – therefore set your standards quickly to avoid set-ups with wasters and no-hopers. Advise if you particularly like or dislike the following: dwarves, ex-cons, hairy gorillas, gingers, DJs, Scotsmen, the visually impaired, Essex boys, Seventies throwbacks, film buffs or train-spotters before you find yourself in a bar with one of them.

Love's secret language

When you agree to meet up with someone the agency says is 'an environmental consultant with his own property in the country and a great sense of humour' there's a good chance you could be about to meet a bin man who takes his holidays in a caravan. Here's a guide to the truth behind the words:

- GSOH = Good sense of humour. However, a good sense of humour can also mean a tendency to make inappropriate jokes in public. Not quite so funny.

- Financially astute = Tight.

- Good looking = Vain.

- Laid back = A dirty slob.

- Cuddly = Fat.

- Free-spirited = A gambler.

- Sociable = A boozer.

- Looking for a casual relationship = Wants to shag other women.

- Enjoys weekends in the country = He doesn't want to introduce you to his friends.

- Works late = Unable to commit to normal dating hours or the wife will find out.

- Open-minded = He would like to try anal sex, three-in-a-bed and sadomasochism.

- Keen = A virgin.

- Creative = Unemployed.

- ◆ Romantic = He's been married four times already.

- ◆ Plays the piano = Badly.

Damage limitation

If possible, get the agency to sift through the thousands of replies on your behalf and send you the cream of the crop. Ten men are enough to be getting on with for any career girl. When you arrange to meet, expect to be disappointed. After all, we all glamorise ourselves don't we? You said you were a natural blonde didn't you? Yeah right – you get my drift. If you're worried about the standard of man the agency can find, ask for a money-back guarantee. I don't mean a confirmation of marriage, just a successful date with someone who doesn't resemble Chewbacca from *Star Wars*. If you are worried about standards, check out the agency's credentials beforehand. Perhaps use one that a friend has recommended, or has a good reputation locally.

Five-question checklist

1. Ask them about success rates – interview them as they interview you.

2. Ask how many couples have got married.

3. Ask how long they continue to search on your behalf.

4. Ask the size of their client base.

5. Ask why they do or why they don't advertise.

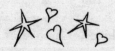

The American dream

Dating agencies in the US are much more forthright about getting the dream partner for their client. Agencies have been set up to fix up ordinary people with models, or at least the very beautiful. Because many people have been put off by agencies, thinking they are the last refuge for ugly desperadoes, some agencies have gone so far as to recruit dates rather than waiting to be approached. They scour top restaurants, trendy bars, acting colleges and model agencies to find dream dates for their clients.

NB Meet a man, not an escort. Make sure you are approaching the right kind of agency. You don't want to enjoy a successful date and be confronted by an invoice and a sexual invitation at midnight. Personal agencies offer sex, pure and simple. Dating agencies offer dates, with the incentive of sex.

Love's wide web

Internet dating has got to be the easiest form of speculative matchmaking – except when you accidentally start flirting with someone on the other side of the world and by the time you've realised it, you're smitten. But Internet dating can also be cheap, quick and safe so long as you're careful. It can offer safe flirting with a large group of people – you'll have access to more men than you would get through a dating ad or agency. You could meet like-minded people too, men in the same boat as you who also don't fancy trailing around bars looking for a shag or people too busy in their professional lives to maintain the normal rules of dating and socialising. Get over the fact that not all users of Internet dating services are morris-dancing computer geeks! You're on the web and you're not sad. So chances are that they aren't either. Get over it.

Internet guidelines

You cannot completely trust someone you've been chatting to on the Internet until you've met them or at least had a few phone conversations. When you first decide to 'cyber-date', follow these safety guidelines:

◆ Take things slowly and don't disclose any private information such as your home or mobile phone number, work/home address or bra size (you could attract perverts).

◆ Even giving out your email address could be a bit dodgy – so why not set up a new account as a safeguard.

◆ Get as much information as possible straight away: age, occupation, nationality, family, and past relationships. You could even ask for some photographs. Of course, you can't guarantee that a stranger at the other end of your modem is telling you the truth, so if you pick up on any fishy vibes or contradictions get out of there.

◆ If he's extra keen to meet up straight away, be careful. You may write to this guy but you don't know him. Spend longer in your computer communication and you'll get more of a feel for his real motivations. Remember the Internet is prime hunting ground for perverts and the sexually bizarre so you can never be too careful.

Saying all this, many great people use the Internet to find love but if you do arrange to meet up, make sure it's in a public place, i.e. a busy bar or restaurant in an area you know well. Tell a family member or friend what you're doing, who you're going with and where you're going. Never invite your prospective date back to your house, or go back to his. This can be said for any first dates, not just the Internet variety. And never get into a car with a stranger – however normal he seems. If he's a decent bloke he'll more than understand.

MELISSA, 30

❝ I had been on an Internet dating site for two months and had gone out on about six dates and met many total weirdos and no Mr Rights. I later realised that my problem probably stemmed from my code name. You have to make up a name (not your real one) that you'll be known as on the site. Now I grew up on the New Jersey shore in America so decided I'd call myself 'Shorething'. I thought it was a witty pun and would show that despite being intelligent and professional I had a sense of humour. Well unfortunately, I think most people took it as a blatant claim to promiscuity and I got mails such as: 'Hi, my name is David. I'm a young (19 years) inexperienced man and have something about older women. Basically I'm looking for an older woman to teach me something about the female body (sex). So if you're up for a hot dirty time with a younger man then please contact me. And who knows maybe if we like each other we can go for a long-term relationship.' Afterwards, I laughed hysterically and tried not to be shocked that at 29 I'd reached the older-woman status. Luckily before my Internet time ran out I met Duncan, who is wonderful, and we're still together. My advice would be don't get disheartened by freaks and fools. ❞

Distant flirtations

Once you've got a bit of a thing going with someone from an Internet dating site or have swapped email addresses with a friend's friend, you can if you wish make things a bit more intimate. Now is the time to learn how to email... and I don't mean the kind you send to your best friend to confirm cocktails or to the secretary you can't stand two desks down. I mean a sexy, or at least romantic, email. Email is good because you can flirt shamelessly knowing that you won't have to face the possibility that your date might take you up on your offers, you can develop nervous twitches and blush and he'll never know, and you can entertain yourself at work on a dull afternoon.

'E-male' rules

1. You shouldn't get too carried away and promise him too much because he may hold you to it when you do finally meet.

2. Remember that companies do check email content for swear words, state secrets and porn so don't email anything you wouldn't want your lawyer to know about you.

3. Handwritten letters are more romantic than a bleep in your inbox, but hey, we're busy people. Email can speed up the love process; just make sure you don't get carried away over a man you've only typed to. And remember, length is pivotal. Just because it's computerised doesn't mean it can't be soppy... and last for over two screens.

4. He writes a good line, but what does he sound like? Before you get too into your emailing relationship, pick up the phone to check out his voice. You'll both be

nervous… what is it about modern people who can discuss their sex lives in front of millions of Jerry Springer fans but hate one-to-one intimacy? Phone on your mobile, because then you can have the excuse of poor reception, high winds and tunnels if the conversation is a non-starter. If you like his voice and the chit-chat goes quite breezily – with both of you making an effort – think about meeting up for a first date.

5. You can make social plans via email, but you shouldn't really cancel them in this way. That's rude and dismissive.

6. Never dump someone via email. Even if you can't bear to look at his smug, arrogant face again, pick up the phone. It won't sound sincere via email, and the tone can easily be misconstrued. It's also hard evidence for him to wave round the pub when he wants sympathy for going out with a bitch.

7. Be funny but not too weird. If friends have warned you that you have a sarcastic, ironic or wacky sense of humour which can be taken the wrong way (you come across either as a vicious queen, a clever clogs or a simpleton) calm it down until you've actually spoken to your virtual date and they know how to take you.

8. Send one email, and then wait for the reply. Don't get clingy and post gentle reminders that you're waiting for a new mail every 20 minutes. He could be busy, in a meeting… he could be on the toilet for God's sake; you know what men are like. There's nothing worse than a desperate email to really put someone off you. When you get an email from him, don't reply within three seconds if you're trying to play it cool.

9. Don't forward his saucy or romantic emails to your friends. Just because you've got them written down, that doesn't mean you can lend them out like a book at a library. They're private.

10. Don't get upset if you find out you're not the only one he's been emailing. Email isn't a marriage certificate, however intimate the contents get. Only feel possessive if you've chatted on the phone a few times or actually met up.

Email stalking

Do not start flirtatiously emailing someone if you have got their address through improper means. You can virtually date if you've been fixed up by a dating agency, friends, or met once and swapped addresses. You should never find email addresses in magazines, company contacts books or on business websites and pester someone.

Here is a date request that gets into dodgy stalking-like behaviour. This is an email sent to a journalist friend of mine from an admiring reader who wanted to do a little more than congratulate her on her work.

Dear Deirdre,

I am one of your fancy that enjoys your column in Woman's Own magazine here in Nigeria & I commend you for a job well done, keep it up and I luv you.†I'd like to adopt you as my sister because I really luv you & if not you have married, I would have luv to marry you. Am a guy that have been dreaming to have a lady from Europe as a wife but due inability to travel my dream yet to come true. I want you to match me with a lady, she may be one of your friends or a lady from Scotland, England,

Holland, Australia, Denmark, US, Sweden & Germany. I know
that you don't enter into personal correspondence, but you can
do it for me for the shake of God & luv. Match me with a lady.
I will be glad if my request can be considered.

Segun

And she was on the first plane to Nigeria – no seriously.
This is clearly not the way forward for this desperate young
man, or for that matter my colleague. Doesn't he know
there are websites for this kind of thing? Needless to say,
email someone out of bounds and you too could look this
daft. Think before you type.

Text before marriage?

A further sign of our twenty-first-century refusal to go on
normal dates is the craze for text-dating that's sweeping...
well, not the world, more like busy PR girls living in busy
cities. Texting a prospective date is fun because you have
complete control – you can choose whether you respond, or
avoid messages by turning off your phone. So all round
great news for hard-working socialites like us, right? Err,
well, maybe not. The first problem is remembering to keep
your charger with you at all times. You don't want a dead
battery to come between you and the man of your dreams.
This may sound simple but can be easily forgotten amongst
gym bags and briefcases. Text-dating is good in cold
weather but a bit boring if you're sociable. Basically all you
need to indulge in text-dating is a mobile and a brain. Talking of which, mobiles apparently fry your mind if you use
them too much.

So how do you actually meet a man via a phone line? Firstly you sign up to a text-dating agency, found on the Internet. At some agencies, for example, you hand over the joining fee, answer a few questions about yourself and give them your mobile number and they promise to get you a few text dates within a week. The next stage of text-dating is that either you start writing to your date and seeing if you get on, or the agency will text you and your unknown date the same message with a time and a place to meet. It's a very secret service which can be quite exciting... but a bit crap if messages get lost, or sent to the wrong number, and you're left in a bar looking like a lemon all night, clutching your mobile phone. Perhaps not the most productive dating method but fun for the very modern among you who want to try everything. Again, don't give out personal information.

Speed-dating

This is all about time, obviously. We want men and we want them now. Trouble is we're busy. So can we meet ten eligible bachelors at the same time please? Why of course! Dating is a big industry where all needs are taken care of, hence the growth in special dating events.

Below are a few examples of high-octane flirting events, which may seem a bit predatory. But if 100 single people in a room know what they're looking for, at least they're with like-minded available dudes rather than the married or the resolute commitment-phobes.

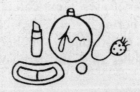

Where do you go to my lovely?

Introduction agencies

These agencies are a good place to start looking for speed-dating events. For people who are unsure about going on one-on-one dates, they often set up casual cocktail parties where their clients can meet each other. This means you can take a friend along for moral support – and fix her up at the same time.

Supermarkets

Singles shopping nights in supermarkets have been marketed as a bit of a dating coup. I always thought it was an urban myth that a couple really fell in love when their eyes met over the frozen peas but it does happen. Contact the head offices of the larger supermarket chains, or if you're brave enough, suggest it at your local branch. After all: 'If music be the food of love...' why not have suggestive conversations at the sausage meat counter while listening to the pan-pipe sounds of the Seventies?

Singles holidays

Singles holidays (brochures can be found at any travel agent's) are good for people who are looking for love, or just want to get away from all the other smug marrieds you see moping together over the hotel salad bar. The obvious bonus is that you're not at work so you will feel more relaxed, and this allows you to meet people you wouldn't normally give the time of day to. Hopefully you've chosen somewhere warm so you'll have a great tan and be feeling more attractive. And you don't have to set up dates or book cabs – you're in the same place!

One-off events

Specially organised one-off events haul in hundreds of dateless young things. After all, with eight million single people in the UK, they've got to go somewhere. Often they are themed balls or weekends away, offering masses of snog-inducing free beer once you've paid the upfront price. These things can soon degenerate into meat markets... you're all pissed and all looking for a bit of a grope. Don't go to one of these if you're looking for true love, you'll be lucky to find it while you're queuing for the loo. But do go if you're looking for a bit of 'physical intimacy' as my mum would say.

Evening all

Evening classes aren't set up as a hotbed of passion and romance, but pick your courses carefully and you can find true love while learning how to wire a plug. Obviously, don't sign up to flower-arranging, needlework, childcare or cake-baking, as not many men attend. Try general courses like photography, painting and French, or the full-macho, high-testosterone car-maintenance workshop or plumbing. The men will think you're cool and interesting – and you'll already have something in common so starting conversations should be easy. After a few months, suggest a trip to the pub to discuss coursework, or hint that a Christmas party for the class could be a real laugh. Smarm up to the tutor (not in an OTT class sucker way) so that he always makes you sound fabulously intelligent and goes along with any social suggestions you might make.

This kind of dating is all about self-autonomy – you go get 'em, girl. However confident you become you should not overcompensate and start looking for love under any unturned stone you come across. Places that should, generally, be avoided at all costs include:

- ◆ Prisons: The prison welfare service encourages relationships with the outside world but be careful. They are under no obligation to tell you about their crimes and it's in the prisoner's interest to lie to any women who come their way. Women have been known to fall in love through the bars, get married before their husband is released, and then be murdered when he leaves jail in a situation spookily similar to his previous crime. Try the non-convicted first. You get more sex with a free man if nothing else.

- ◆ Rehab centres: However much of a help-all nature you have, they need to help themselves first. Get back to that evening class to pass your spare time.

- ◆ Moaning meetings: Don't go to those single-mother, hate-men, hate-married-people, hate-being-divorced, hate-being-single clubs, or similar. They're bitter and it will rub off on you. Yep, everyone knows you're single and miserable about it so be proactive not dogmatic.

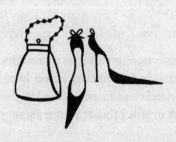

Secrets of Success

◆ Don't panic. Although it can get lonely and depressing at times, you're not alone. There are millions of fish in the sea, plenty enough for everyone.

◆ Don't think you're sad or desperate for outsourcing your dating needs. Modern girls outsource their cleaning, gardening, work administration – we even hire personal trainers to take care of our bodies so we don't have to. Employing an agency is an extension of sharing the load. Let the experts find the right man for you, or at least tell you where to look.

◆ Leave out the personal details. However great someone sounds, don't be too trusting. It's a cynical view but could stop you being stalked by an unwanted admirer.

◆ Try to be honest about yourself. If you're a 5 ft brunette don't post a picture of a 6 ft blonde on your website. If things kick off, you'll get found out and look stupid.

◆ Don't believe the hype. Just because you're acting with decorum and telling the truth, it doesn't mean your fellow singletons are. Always treat their websites and emails with a healthy distrust. Don't turn into a paranoid psycho though.

◆ Give it time. The people running dating agencies and websites are professionals, not miracle workers. You can't have a 'paid my cash, where's my man' attitude. It's almost better if they don't rush you into lots of dodgy dates.

◆ Check out your dating medium thoroughly. Don't sign up or pass over cash to businesses found in phone booths or on flyers. Ask friends, research on the Internet and ask them to send you full details of what you're signing up to.

◆ Pick a reasonable pseudonym. Pussy Galore could sound too forward; Plain Jane could be a bit off-putting. You don't want to put prospective dates off but you don't want to come across as a harlot either.

◆ Don't send porn as an incentive.

◆ But do try phone, email, or text sex with someone you like the sound of... it's the safest form out there – diseases aren't carried on airwaves. As long as you can get over the initial embarrassment of telling a stranger about your fiddly bits. Let's face it, this encounter may be more erotic than when you see him face-to-face and he turns out to be a spotty dwarf.

◆ Avoid premium-rate dating phone lines and singles chat rooms on the Internet. You'll meet perverts and simpletons – and waste money in the process. The only person getting regular sex on these lines is the owner who's stinging you for cash and flashing it for the ladies in the Canaries.

◆ Equally avoidable should be the psychic phone lines – I doubt a hard-up housewife in Hull can predict your future husband any more than you could.

◆ Do make a public display of yourself and go on one of the many new dating shows. You'll get your make-up and hair done and the television researchers will do all the work for you. As long as you don't mind the world knowing if you're a bad kisser...

◆ Think carefully before you fill out a dating agency application form. One slip of the pen and you could be fixed up with a pensioner and not a television commissioner.

◆ When leaving a phone message for your dial-a-date, speak clearly and slowly. Rush through your words with a breathy gasp and he'll think you're a bit too erotically charged.

◆ If you're sensible, you'll avoid looking for love at your school reunion. You can't have your first passionate encounter 30 years after you showed him your knickers in the playground. There's too much history there, and besides the Head may try to make you appear in the local paper as a 'local celebrity couple' to promote the school fun run (two words that I never thought went together).

◆ If you are serious about pulling, hang out with other single people of the same sexual persuasion as you – you'll never get hot hetero action in a gay bar.

◆ Don't get depressed if it all seems a bit crazy. Remember, this is the best decade ever to be single. In the 1940s and 1950s, you were given one strike at love then out; in the 1960s everyone was too stoned or busy throwing knickers at pop stars to have a proper relationship. In the 1970s, you just wouldn't, would you? And, in the 1980s, unless you met someone in your high-powered office, you couldn't get near another single person for his or her huge shoulder pads and brick-like mobile phones. In the 1990s, we were all just a little too politically correct. Now, however, we say and feel what we want. Modern technology is at our fingertips to find us a date. Wahoo!

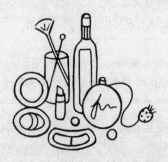

Chapter Four

Do-it-yourself

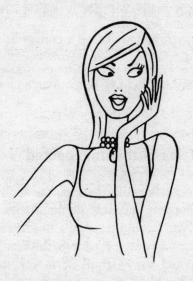

MODERN GIRLS ARE sassy, sexy and self-assured... so perhaps they don't need to rely on friends, family and professional fixers to find a date? Often it's a case of recognising opportunities when they come your way – and knowing what to do with them.

Distant friends

Although it's good to have the instant approval of your comrades, it's sometimes good to bump into a prospective date without the opinion of your friends, family or a professional.

- *En masse* you are harder to approach.

- In company, you may be missing opportunities.

- Your friends could take the mickey out of your flirting technique...

- ...Or put you off a perfectly decent chap for the fun of it.

- On your own, you can strike up a conversation without being observed.

- And no one will be there to tell embarrassing stories to the new man.

Tales of the unexpected

For once, you're not actually looking for a love interest. You're going about your business, getting things done when – wham bam – Mr 'I could pass as a Brad Pitt impersonator' stumbles across your everyday path. You feel like an overfed baboon and the yoghurt stain on your shirt is screaming 'dirty scrubber' so you can't believe it when he catches your eye and smiles. Here's how to cope with unexpected flirtations:

- Smile back briefly, and as spontaneously as you can – not like a simpleton.

- Don't look shocked, point at your chest, and mouth: 'What, me?' when he makes eyes at you.

- Don't rush to the nearest mirror to check your appearance before you indulge in some flirting. You don't normally walk around with spinach between your teeth or your skirt caught in your knickers, so you can be 99.9% sure you're not now.

- Don't rush straight over – indulge in a few minutes of silent flirting (using eyes, smiles and body language – more on this is in chapter 5) until one of you feels ready to make a move. It's more difficult making the first move in an unexpected environment, without the dating props of alcohol and dim lighting.

- If you're passing in the street or on an escalator and time is more urgent, you can turn on your heel and chase if you are feeling supremely confident and don't mind an audience. Passers-by will know what you're up to so you have to prepare yourself for humiliation.

- Don't panic if you blush. Worrying about blushing normally makes you blush more. Instead do the whole bowed-head, hair-flicking shy look men find attractive.

- Don't freak out and run away or hide if he approaches you. Be still your feet!

- If you can't stop shaking or fidgeting while he's making his way over, suddenly take great interest in your handbag, book or diary. This will take your mind off his imminent arrival.

- If you can't think of anything interesting to say at first, fall back on the old classic – the weather conversation, especially if you're outside.

- Don't worry about acting cool. Feel free to comment on how weird the situation is.

- Use the environment to make conversation – ask him what he's buying, drinking, or planning on doing?

- Find out if 'he comes here often'. If he does, the pressure is off to swap details immediately – just expect to hang around this location more than usual... which is good if it's your gym, but bad if it's the smelly recycling plant ten miles from your house.

VANESSA, 31

❝ I saw this stunning man at my doctor's surgery. He obviously had a heavy cold and we smiled sympathetically at each other through our sniffles. When the receptionist came around to apologise for the delay – we'd both been kept waiting ages – he used the time dilemma as an excuse to chat. Pretending to need a new magazine, I walked over to the stack, which was helpfully positioned next to him, to get a better look. We swapped cold cures, basic info about each other and then arranged to meet in the coffee shop next to the chemist after we picked up our prescriptions. Not the most romantic of meetings, and I only saw him a few times, but it goes to show you can meet someone at any time. ❞

Novel love locations

Gym or health club

This is great. Gym memberships are so expensive you have to go at least twice a week to justify the cost and you're likely to bump into him again. It also means he's likely to care about his appearance, be quite fit and very clean (gymgoers take regular showers). Hopefully he's not the vain Arnie-type who looks at himself in the mirror while lifting weights.

When to approach
Take a trip to the water cooler when he does, or follow him into the sauna for a relaxing steam. Don't interrupt during an exercise class, circuits, or an underwater swim. Tapping on his shoulder when he's about to dive into the pool will frustrate him and possibly harm you (flying legs and arms everywhere).

What to say
Comment on the new fitness instructor, the parking (men love any excuse to talk about cars generally). You could even comment on your aching muscles (this may draw his eye to affected areas, make him think you train hard, and he might even fantasise about giving you a massage).

Bus stop or train station

It may be difficult to concentrate on the cute guy grinning at you when you're worried about being late for work, but love waits for no man. A bit of flirting can help pass the time when waiting for your preferred mode of transport. Again, seeing him at your bus stop – especially on a work-day – is good because he probably uses the route regularly. Yippee – you'll see him again!

When to approach
Other than praying the only empty seat is next to you, make small talk in an informal, friendly manner while queuing. It could be too early in the morning to indulge in full-on flirting (lots of people don't wake up until they've had a coffee at their desk). Make sure you always get in the queue at the same time each day. If he likes you, he'll make sure he's there too.

What to say

Pray for freak circumstances (bad rain, bad roadworks or a heatwave) to bring you together. Find out where he gets off – this will lead easily into questions about where he works and lives, which will promote further small talk.

Coffee, or lunch-break hangout

Bumping into a potential date while you're at work can bring a little joy to your day. It can also make Monday mornings a lot easier to cope with. You'll also become popular with colleagues who can't believe you're so keen to do all the tea-runs. Chances are you'll be with a work mate during your breaks, so you can also get a quick second opinion – is he really sexy? Does he look interested?

When to approach

Linger around the crisp counter until he gets in the queue, and then nab the spot behind him. Ask him to pass you an apple when your hands are full and feel free to explain that the 12 chocolate bars aren't all for you, you're treating your department (you'll look generous and fun).

What to say

After bumping into him more than three times, start saying hello and ask him what he's having. Under no circumstances say: 'Coffee, tea, me?' Do ask him if he drinks in any of the bars around your office.

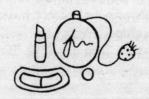

Supermarket

People don't normally get dolled up to go food shopping, so if he's throwing out a few positive signals now, he thinks you're dynamite. Try and get a good look in his supermarket trolley: you may be able to detect if he lives on his own, is a vegetarian, has a healthy, balanced diet and appreciates chocolate as much as you do.

When to approach

Certainly don't sidle over when he's looking at an embarrassing counter (contraceptives, toilet tissues and pickled-onion displays are all out for your first romantic encounter). Search for a neutral area – the frozen vegetables are always a good bet. Trolleys are infamously free-spirited so plan a mini-collision.

What to say

Don't go for foodie double entendres. Despite your locations, jokes about marrows, cucumbers, and meat and two veg are never acceptable (except on girls-only office parties). Go for the subtle: 'Do you know where the light bulbs are?' If you get chatting, suggest having a coffee in the supermarket café. Play it down by saying you need some caffeine or you're addicted to the doughnuts and you're always collaring strangers to come with you.

Shops

Browsing in a music, book or clothes shop is good. It means he's not in a rush to get anywhere. It also gives you the chance to judge his style and think of conversation-openers. Avoid a man hanging out in a lingerie or women's clothes shop – he either has a girlfriend already or he's a pervert.

This situation is a bit more urgent however; he may not be back there for months, if not ever!

When to approach

Subtly move around the aisles so he can see you in the distance before suddenly (how did you do that!) finding yourself standing side-by-side at an interesting display. Pick up the same book, CD, or whatever – catch his eye and make an interesting comment about the author (if a book) for example, and ask him a question – he'll be forced to respond.

What to say

'I love this book!' 'Do you know where *blah blah* is or when it's coming out?' Ask his advice – men like to feel knowledgeable and needed. Go with the flow. The great thing about meeting in a shop is that there is a wealth of interesting props around and unless you're making your move in the January sales, there will be many chances to break off from the crowd.

How to ask for a date without asking

If you can't pluck up the courage to ask him out and haven't got the patience to wait for him, there are a number of handy hints you can drop to make your intentions obvious:

◆ Ask him when he's next going to be working out, shopping or travelling and say you hope to see him again soon.

◆ Find out how he gets to and from the 'meeting place' – you could offer him a lift next time if he gets the bus etc.

◆ If you've met in a group environment, suggest you all get together in a few weeks for a drink.

◆ Tell him about any social events the college, gym, or restaurant are holding over the next few weeks and let him know you're interested in going.

◆ Get the conversation round to the weekend, and jokingly complain that all your friends have turned really boring since getting into relationships, and if you're not careful the only relationship you'll have on a Friday night is with your remote control. If he's interested and chivalrous, he'll think about saving you from this fate.

Looking inconspicuous

There's nothing worse than a girl looking like a fish out of water, sipping on a glass of champagne amongst a group of beer-swilling, song-chanting football supporters. You have to look like you belong or it will be obvious why you're there – not to relax, chat, drink or dance, but to pull. The wrong kind of man will think: 'Superb, she's up for it, why else is she here?' The right kind of guy will think: 'How weird, doesn't she have any interests/friends of her own?', unless your natural charms are so overwhelming he falls for you despite your Eliza Doolittle impression in the Ascot Private Members enclosure.

Maybe you should adopt a disguise and adjust your sensibilities. I'm not talking about a plastic mac, Cleopatra wig or sunglasses. I mean only going to places where you have some natural affiliation and dressing appropriately. It would be a bit odd to suddenly take up golf after years of hating the game, simply in order to spend more time at the 19th hole with the dishy pro. No, that's not the way forward. If you and your friends have always enjoyed watching rugby on television, go to a pub and watch it there instead – wearing sensible clothes and not the new minidress and stilettos you bought for your sister's hen night. You'll get attention but almost certainly the wrong kind. If you work in a bank, start going out socially with your colleagues rather than rushing home to wash your hair. Just learn to draw a line between work banter and work gossip.

Where not to go on the prowl

Gay clubs

So the music might be better and the sequin count may be higher but understand that the men are gay. They are *not* interested. You can't change their minds. Yes they're prettier, cooler and you have more in common but ultimately they won't shag you and what's the use in that?

Prison

Loving someone on the inside may make you feel like a martyr. Helping someone in need brings out the maternal instinct in lots of girls. But (apart from exceptional circumstances), if he's in prison, he's bad. Let's face it – the fact he's locked up at Her Majesty's Pleasure gives you the most wonderful insight into his personality.

Rehab clinics

Addiction is a problem for lots of people and before they can nurture a relationship, they need to look after themselves. Unless you're already emotionally involved with an addict, it's probably better to avoid dating a gambler, drug abuser or alcoholic until they've got their own heads straight. They'll only mess up yours.

Tasmania

Avoid back-of-beyond places where the men outnumber the women by 10:1. However cute the guys look in their plaid shirts, the story will be very different when you've packed up and shipped out to the middle of nowhere. Get to know him in both environments before you commit to a life of farming and early nights.

Parents' parties

Well, it's just creepy, isn't it? Monica in *Friends* managed to make dating her parents' friend chic for about, erm, two seconds. And then the world woke up. It's pervy. They think the same, go to the same places and enjoy the company of the people who've most likely embarrassed you more than anyone else. You don't so leave it there.

Boss's office

Unless there are exceptional circumstances, i.e. your boss looks like George Clooney, has the wealth of Richard Branson and has offered to relocate you to a dream job if you sleep with him, try to avoid stalking him at your office. Especially while actually at work. If you've weighed up the consequences, fancy your chances, and have had a bit to drink at the office Christmas party, go for it. First-date sex on his desk shouldn't be an option, however, especially if he's married.

Club 18-30 holidays

These holidays are a good laugh but you're not going to find the man of your dreams sidling up to you over a tequila and wet T-shirt competition. Go with your girlfriends and have a few snogging competitions, just don't get your hopes up that one of your victims will become long-term. It may happen but the odds are against you.

A train-spotters' convention

Well, unless you want to be bored to death. Enough said?

Legions of foreign men

If you feel confident looking for a mate on your own, why not take yourself off to foreign climes where matchmaking has become an industry. It makes sense – the chances of bumping into someone you know will lessen, you'll be able to pick up cheap perfume at the Duty Free and if you meet a few nightmares, you can fly home safe in the knowledge they won't be following you.

Alaska

Okay, so the men are little bit beardy and their idea of high-fashion daywear is a plaid shirt and a husky on a lead, but if you're desperate... there are thousands of them waiting for your visit. Each December, the eligible bachelors of Talkeetna (just outside state capital Anchorage) are sold to female bidders in a dating auction. The newly formed couples then get to know each other over a week of wood-chopping, pint-pouring and snow-shovelling.

Australia

Limited to singletons aged between 18–35, the Saturday night before Valentine's Day is officially for the D&D's – the desperate and dateless. All those who want to attend the official balls give the organisers their details, and a date is arranged for them. Thousands of people attend so if you're into Aussie hunks, you're sorted. It's in aid of the Red Cross so at least you're helping charity in your pursuit of love.

Germany

This is a tough one but desperate times call for desperate measures. It's tradition in Hanover that all men must sweep the Town Hall's steps on their 30th birthday, so linger about there and you're bound to pick up a youngish man with good domestic skills eventually.

Ireland

The Lisdoonvarna Matchmaking Festival is possibly the most popular singles holiday in the world. Every year, the small town comes alive with people on the love lookout. Dances, drinks and days in the local beautifying spas are laid on, and the Queen of *Blind Date* herself – our Cilla – is reputed to be a fan.

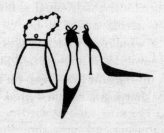

Sardinia

Singles-only dinner dates on this beautiful island can't fail to succeed. A few glasses of Chianti and a suck on some spaghetti and you're bound to find love. Many holiday companies arrange large events which are advertised on the Internet and in specialist brochures.

> ### EMMA, 30
>
> ❝ I needed a bit of R&R (rest & relaxation) and all my friends were shacked up and saving so didn't fancy a girls' holiday. I thought a singles break would be good not so much because I wanted to find a boyfriend but because I didn't want to be surrounded by mushy couples groping each other in the swimming pool. I love Italian food, history and wine so decided to go to Sardinia. Even though I didn't find my future husband, I met lots of interesting people who I would never normally meet... and had a laugh listening to the other single girl's dating stories. ❞

Seattle

You might be sleepless, but from too much shagging rather than panic attacks. The city of shrinks has developed its own self-help cure for the sadly singles. Eight-minute dating has been set up across many of the city's bars and hot nightspots. Each woman is matched with eight men, who then have eight minutes to impress her. How perfect – you can get the full, no-bullshit low-down on the man and then disappear pretty sharpish if he's not what you're after.

Secrets of Success

◆ Keep an eye out for tasty men 24/7... but be subtle. Remember to have a life at the same time. Don't prowl the streets with your tongue hanging out.

◆ In case of an unexpected meeting, maintain a certain level of grooming. Don't make a habit of going out wearing stained clothes, laddered tights or shell suits. Try to keep hair, nails and armpits clean and fresh.

◆ Practise applying bronzing powder and lip-gloss in extreme, rushed conditions (always keep them in your bag) in case of emergencies.

◆ Instead of panicking that you're on your own, let your independence liberate you to become a more self-assured, confident version of the you your friends and family know.

◆ Don't underestimate honesty — if you really like him, approach him. If he laughs or walks away, comfort yourself with the fact you'll probably never see him again.

◆ When sharking on your own, take extra care. Never give out your home address or phone number. It's better to arrange to meet somewhere there and then or swap email addresses. Do not go to their home or get in a car with them. A decent guy will understand why.

◆ Keep your diary on you to make arrangements.

◆ Even if the man made the first move — striking up a conversation or smiling — he may be too nervous to actually ask you out. Feel free to take the bull by the horns. If his body language is saying he likes you, he'll be grateful.

◆ Use your senses – is he looking at you, smiling at you, how is his voice? Watch out for the signs and feel the vibes.

◆ Don't feel embarrassed about going on singles holidays. They are very, very popular and provide a relaxed, neutral environment for people to meet new people.

◆ Don't let the sun, sea and sangria (or such substances) warp your judgement. Have a flirt, kiss, or whatever... but don't let the holiday spirit get to your heart or your wallet too quickly.

◆ If you met someone on your own, keep it between the two of you for a while. Allow the relationship to develop slowly before you bring in external factors like drunken colleagues and an overbearing mother.

Chapter Five

How to be irresistible

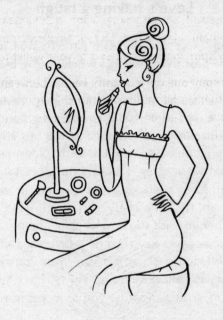

WE ALL HAVE GOOD days and bad days and when you're single, these matter. You never know when Mr Gorgeous is going to be around the corner. For the purpose of pulling alone, one should try to maintain at least a minimum standard of grooming at all times. I'm not suggesting you turn into a pampered human poodle that can't leave the house without at least two hours of cosmetic preparation. No one likes high-maintenance women – they are frustrating, time-consuming and men automatically assume a negative correlation between the amount of hair lacquer used and your brain cells. What I am suggesting is working on your good bits – and forgiving your bad bits – so you feel confident, attractive and ready for action – whenever it may strike.

Love's having a laugh

We've already accepted that the path to true love isn't a smooth one – just like your legs when you've unexpectedly met the man of your dreams only to have him sexily stroke two chimp-like limbs under the table. It seems to be love's unwritten rule that when you do bump into a potential date on a night out with your friends, at the bus stop, or in a meeting, you *will* have greasy hair with bad roots, be wearing thousand-wash grey knickers in a certain state of disrepair and have a beacon-sized spot on the end of your nose. These are the little challenges that life likes to throw at us. So either go with the flow or take comfort in the fact that if he fancies you like this, he'll be insatiable once he's seen you dolled up. Or make sure you constantly wear matching, newish underwear and always have 'just stepped out of a salon' tresses. Because you're worth it, remember?

What do men find attractive?

This is impossible to answer – just as some women go for skinny geeks and others go for muscle-bound beefcakes, men have widely varying tastes. Different strokes for different folks, as the saying goes. And if you want to have some strokes, you better find your niche. So don't get despondent if you keep fancying men who go for blonde waifs and you're a curvy brunette. If we all went for the same thing, life would be very dull indeed. Respect the fundamentals: everyone likes a basic level of cleanliness but, apart from that, feel free to plough your own furrow on the looks front.

Dress to impress

Because everyone has his or her own idea of what's attractive, I'd say dress to suit you not a potential date. You might suspect your dream man is a stiletto and suspender fetishist but if it means you walking like a crab on your first date, forget it. Plump for the trainers and cotton knickers. You'll be able to get your round in at the bar without scaring him and feel a lot more comfortable to boot.

Undercover story

Certain items of clothing will win you favour with men, so as long as you feel comfortable it could be worth experimenting with them:

- Stilettos: Basically high heels of any description. Not only do they elongate the leg but, psychologists say, they give the foot the same shape it assumes when a woman orgasms. Interesting. Stilettos are associated with feminine power, glamour and, yes, kinky sex and this may be more to the point. Men are essentially perverts with dominatrix fantasies.

- Sexy underwear: There are a few men who prefer the clean and white variety of undergarments but the immoral majority like lacy bits of cheese wire in red and black. It's amazing how much sexier you feel knowing you look great underneath your clothes. Donning a pair of lacy stockings and hold-ups will make you feel more confident on a manhunt than a pair of tummy-tuck tights. Some may argue that peephole bras and crotchless knickers in waterproof fabrics are even more erotic. I'd say they're a bit too much.

♦ Glasses: Yep, that's right. Spectacles *can* be sexy. If you're meeting for a date straight from work, keep them on to achieve that seductive-secretary-turned-vamp appeal. Even if you are the MD of the company.

♦ Miniskirts: Men aren't subtle and they like to sample the menu before they order, so if you've got great pins, get them out.

♦ Any top that shows ample cleavage: Whether it's something to do with being breastfed as a baby, or some strange homoerotic arse similarity, men are obsessed with boobs. Having big boobs (speaking from personal experience) means random men are nice to you for no reason. They are more willing to leave their friends and chat to you and your 'two bosom buddies'. Of course, this isn't necessarily a good thing. A girl wants to be appreciated for her brain, but until you've won him over with your outstanding general knowledge, give him more front than Brighton. If you're on the small side, invest in a wonderbra or similar. Toilet-paper stuffing is so 1950s. Oh, the suffragettes will be turning in their graves... Remember, not too much (and certainly no nipples) to avoid looking cheap.

♦ Sports clothing: It's simple, wearing a tracksuit without sweat marks speaks volumes for your energy, enthusiasm and fitness. Men will interpret this one way: great body, good in bed and low maintenance. There is a fine line to tread style-wise so think more J-Lo's dance tracksuits than luminous cycling shorts.

NB Dress for success. Do not try to be cute and appealing on dates by wearing a school uniform, twin-set and pearls, leather catsuit, no knickers, anorak, football shirt or bunny-girl costume. All of the above could be misinterpreted and attract the wrong sorts.

Suit your shape

There's no point going for the male-pleasing uniform of stilettos and miniskirts if you're 6 ft 3 inches and size 20 – you'll look like a transvestite. There are guidelines to follow to make the most of your figure.

Athletic

You lucky madam, you're slim and neatly proportioned. In theory you can get away with anything – regardless of height – but if you want to add curves, wear patterns, never wear the same colour head-to-toe and try asymmetrical tops and skirts. Avoid leggings at all times. Never be ashamed to invest in plump-up bra and chicken-fillet fillers (those breast-shaped plastic bags to slip into your bra).

Petite

Avoid wearing tents and cagoules, or any other clothing made of vast amounts of fabric. They'll swamp you. Wear one shade, this will make you look taller. Show some flesh, it will make you look more proportioned. Avoid over-accessorising, you'll look like a Christmas tree. Wear high heels if you can, a few inches can make a big difference.

Tall

Don't slouch; be proud. Nothing is worse than a tall person walking around like the Hunchback of Notre Dame. Make the most of your long legs with slimming cigarette pants and pencil skirts. You can wear the long, flowing variety of skirts and flares more that any other body shape so give it a go. Wear heels if you want to – don't ever feel you are tall enough already if you fancy a sexy look.

Curvy

Be proud of your womanly shape and emphasise it with fitted, tailored clothes. If you've got big boobs, avoid breast pockets, buttons, patterns and roll-necks and stick to V-necks, bodices and skimming shirts. If you are pear-shaped, wear darker shades on your bottom half. Never wear clothes that are too tight for you: bulges and VPL is *not* a good look. It's better to go up a size and cut out the label than share your choice of knickers with the world.

ANGIE, 29

❝ My life has been revolutionised by the many number of tit-tricks a woman has up her sleeve now. I always felt a little flat because I looked so flat and I assumed – and often saw – men going for the big-boobed over me. I didn't blame them because even I, a heterosexual woman, thought they looked sexier! So now, if I'm going out for the night I wear a push-up bra with jelly extras. I love it. And if I do pull and a man goes in for the grope, I act coy and tell him not yet. So my new boobs probably make me more attractive in two ways. ❞

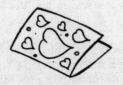

Scents appeal

Some men may argue that natural body odour is a good thing, i.e. 'we don't wash and we've run out of deodorant'. This is true to a degree – fresh out of the shower, women can smell quite pleasant for a while and men for a little less time. But help nature along with some special fragrances – you know it makes scents.

◆ Feeling fruity: Give him a taste of the tropics with some lime, lemon, grapefruit or strawberry cologne or take a long soak in berry-tastic bubble bath.

◆ Musk haves: Search out perfumes with a heady base to bring out the animal instinct.

◆ Floral favourites: Nice and girly for men who like their women to smell like women. Can bring out hay fever in the hypersensitive.

◆ Aftershave: Many women wear men's or unisex fragrances, which can be strong, sexy and powerful.

NB Don't overdo it, a little goes a long way. Your prospective date may like the look of you, adore your dry wit but be allergic to the smell of concentrated lilies. Smell is the most powerful of all the senses, and the one most associated with memory.

As well as choosing a fragrance, keep it clean. Remember cleanliness is next to sex-godliness. If you suffer from smelly feet, spray them with deodorant as well as your armpits before a big night out. If you suffer from halitosis, go to your doctor immediately you unfortunate being (and in the meantime, never leave the house without some chewing gum and a plastic face shield). If you suffer from sweaty palms, forehead, upper lip etc, think about getting an antiperspirant injection. It might not smell like underarm sweat but it can still be embarrassing – and no one should feel self-conscious when looking for love.

NB Fragrant fancies. You've paid a lot of attention to making sure you smell gorgeous so don't make any excuses for men on the pongy side of polite. Okay, we all work hard and we all make mistakes so make a judgement call between fresh sweat and stale sweat. If you suspect the man chatting you up is wearing a day-old shirt, ditch him. Short of pegging your nose while snogging, this relationship is doomed.

Finishing touches

It would be insulting to men to assume that they all like pillar-box red lips and dangerously long talons. Again it's all down to choice. There's the assumption that men like the vamps – the done-up divas that pout through pumped-up lips and gaze seductively through heavy-lidded eyes but some like the natural, fresh look too. Just follow these simple rules...

◆ Avoid the overly made-up look. Men don't like the trowelled-on effect anymore than well-groomed girls do. Ladies who go to bed looking like Elizabeth Hurley and wake up looking like Elizabeth II can warp a man for life. This is where the phrase coyote ugly comes from – men would rather chew off their own arm than stir the transformed lady sleeping at their side (beer goggles can also be blamed for this effect). Wearing lots of make-up also makes it look like you've got something to hide, and unless you have been attacked by a bout of zits it's unnecessary.

◆ Remember every good gay man's catchphrase – make-up should accentuate your natural beauty to look like it is all nature's beauty. Less is more.

◆ Avoid any fluorescent shades and blue mascara. Think about it. The girls in Abba were quite attractive – we just think of them as munters because of their poor taste in make-up.

◆ Blend. Nothing is worse than weird creases and tidemarks around your neck. You'll look like a dirty dog.

◆ Keep top-up products in your handbag (mascara, kohl pencil, concealer, mints and lip-gloss) for emergency re-applications. Don't bring your whole vanity case out on a date though – and keep toilet time to a minimum (you don't want him to think your have diarrhoea).

Hair today, not gone tomorrow

◆ Just keep it clean. Some men think crops are cute, bobs are bold and long hair is seductive, but they're not going to run their fingers through a greasy, tangled mop or kiss a scalp with a gentle dusting of dandruff, no matter how good the cut.

◆ Keep the hair products to a minimum or a rogue lit match could set you burning with the wrong kind of flame. Too much spray will make you look a bit plastic as well – especially if he walks you home and your hair doesn't move an inch during a freak storm.

- Avoid elaborate up-dos which could get caught on light fixtures. These also take a lot of maintaining and you don't want to spend longer in the loos with a selection of hairgrips than with him.

- Fergie bows, cuddly toys on bands and deely-boppers (Alice bands with spring attachments) are never a good idea. Full stop.

Body talk

This pulling thing just gets trickier and trickier... it's not only how you look and smell that attracts the man of your dreams. It's what you say and how you move too. This being a femme fatale business is like spinning plates while sitting on the toilet.

Words of love

A recent survey in a woman's magazine proved that a great personality is the most underrated quality a woman can possess. Sure face, body and sex appeal are all important but if you've got nothing to talk about, what's the point? Men are more like us than we give them credit for. So what do they want from a lady? They like to feel cared for so ask them questions about their career, parents, or friends without appearing too intense. It's a fine line to tread – flatter him into thinking he's interesting without worrying that you'll be asking to see his birth certificate next. I once got chatted up by a famous footballer who was extremely keen until I started telling him stuff about his own life that I'd garnered from his team's official annual. A photographic memory isn't a good thing for a Spurs fan. A girl can know or probe too much.

Another thing to look out for is double-entendres. When a man says: 'Would you like to come up for coffee?' he means: 'Do you fancy a shag?' So do some women but make sure you understand the lingo before you get caught out.

Common misunderstandings

Men

Men say:

- You look beautiful.

- I don't want anything too serious.

- Do you want a drink?

- I don't normally come on this strong.

- I'll call you tomorrow.

Men mean:

- I really, really fancy you.

- Sex please but no questions.

- Buy her a bevvie and she's mine.

- Except every Thursday.

- I'll call you in the acceptable three days.

Women

Women say:

- What, this old thing?

- I love football.

- What do you do for a living?

- Are you still friends with your exes?

- Shall we get a Chinese takeaway?

Women mean:

- Good – he noticed the Gucci.

- I love footballers' legs.

- How much do you earn?

- What's the competition?

- Do you fancy coming to mine for a snog?

The charm defensive

So how do you win a man over in five minutes? By talking about a sport you are genuinely interested in, current affairs you can hold your own in and the musical legacy of The Beatles. Flirt by speaking in a soft voice – no hysterical laughter or shrill exclaiming. Offer him a drink but if he offers to get you one instead, don't refuse. Some men are old-fashioned so save your breath and your money. Ask them questions about themselves and listen to the answers. Pay him genuine compliments – if you don't mean it, zip it. Avoid the subjects of ex-boyfriends, penile implants, politics and cystitis and watch him being reeled in.

Move closer

Now you know what to say, you've got to work that body. Luckily, thousands of experts have studied sexual behaviour so there's no excuse for a girl not to know what's a come-on and what's a come-off-it.

◆ Arm-swinging: Not a good sign, if he can't keep still it means he's desperate to be somewhere else. If he's tapping his fingers too, he's a goner.

◆ Body-bending: Bending the spine away from the person sitting next to you shows dislike, bending backwards conveys immense dislike.

◆ Body-touching: Touching ourselves is seen as quite an erotic act, especially in front of a stranger. I'm not talking about groping your own nether regions, but subconsciously stroking your arm or neck shows what you would like him to be doing to you. He will find this quite a turn-on.

◆ Covering your mouth: Shows you are lacking in confidence.

◆ Crossed arms: Oh so defensive! It may also symbolise nervousness and anxiety. If the elbows are pointing outwards it shows arrogance and self-importance.

◆ Eye contact: If someone holds your gaze for longer than three seconds they are sending you a subconscious sign of honesty and confidence. They like looking into your eyes and want to gauge your reaction to them. Holding eye contact is the biggest giveaway if you fancy someone.

◆ Feet pointing: It's simple – if you like someone, you point your feet towards him or her, if you don't you point your feet in the opposite direction. It's the same with knees – if you sit with your knees almost uncomfortably pointing towards someone, you either fancy them or find them really interesting.

◆ Fiddling with the head or ear: This person is embarrassed by the situation s/he's in.

◆ Flashbulb eye: If someone you are talking to has a sudden, dramatic widening of the eye, watch out. This is a sign of an angry, confrontational character.

◆ Gulping: The up and down motion of the Adam's apple shows stress or embarrassment.

◆ Hands behind the neck: This is a cocky gesture by someone used to being in control.

◆ Hands on hips: Whoever is doing this means business. Elbows out increases the size of the body so you appear larger than normal. The stance gives the impression of imminent action, self-defence and being powerful – but beware if a man does this to you on a date... he considers the person he's talking to inferior to himself.

◆ Head back: You snob – this is a universal sign for superiority and disdain; it's where the expression 'looking down his nose at me' comes from.

◆ Head tilt: A sign of friendliness, interest and concern. Can also show coyness if eyes lowered at same time.

◆ Leaning in towards someone: Obvious – keep talking, honey.

◆ Scratching: Means you disagree with what is being said.

◆ Standing on tiptoes: An attempt to dominate or threaten.

◆ Sticking out tongue: Poking out your whole tongue is a flirty, friendly gesture. Just showing the tip after saying something means you are lying.

◆ Swagger: Upper-body strutting is a sign of confidence – sometimes a bit too much – and a need for attention. Men think it makes them look important, women swagger to appear in control.

◆ Throat-clearing: This is a sign of doubt or disagreement. If someone clears their throat, they are trying to think of how to say something unsavoury or untrue.

◆ Winking: This is a sign of friendliness yet uncertainty. This person wants to be liked.

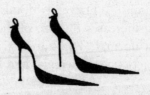

No fun. Period.

A modern girl can groom for va-va-voom to perfection... and still be floored by Mother Nature at the last minute. All girls know getting the decorators in means a possible pimple, a sleepless night, a cramp that doubles you over like a deformed witch (attractive!) and mood swings that scare children and animals at fifty paces.

Of course, I would advise avoiding first dates or any other potentially romantically charged occasions when you're suffering – in case of sudden flood of tears, diarrhoea or leakages – but there is the argument that if girls can skydive and rollerblade on their period, just like all the ads tell us they can, they can charm the pants off a handsome bachelor.

If your diary shows an unfortunate clash, don't make a scene if you can handle it. Just pack enough supplies in your handbag to last you 24 hours (the date may go so well, you end up having breakfast together – not sex necessarily, just a croissant). So make sure you have enough painkillers, tampons, panty liners and clean knickers. An emergency spot cream and concealer could be good too.

> **NB Menstrual facts to remember.** Although it seems unfair, women are increasingly sexually aroused during and straight after their periods. Remember this and don't let your hormones carry you away if it's unwise. Also, it is extremely rare that women get pregnant while they're on but STDs can still get through so still get him to wear a condom. Be aware when drinking and taking painkillers that you'll get drunk much quicker.

Secrets of Success

◆ Get a pulling outfit together. Some things will make you feel sexy, and when you feel sexy, you'll look sexy. If you see an item that suits you, buy it in a few different colours.

◆ Take a trustworthy friend shopping. It's all very well liking the look of something but a friend – of the male variety preferably – can tell you what others will see.

◆ Always check out the back view before you leave the house. You may look great from the front but as you seductively sashay away from your chat-up guy, he may be faced with two hippos wrestling in a sack.

◆ Don't dismiss control underwear until you've tried it. Big knickers can offer wobble-free trips to the bar and confident jiggling on the dance floor. If it does the trick and you pull, you can always swap the pantaloons for a lacy tit-bit in the toilets. Keep something sexy in your handbag if you're worried.

◆ If you're wearing a miniskirt, be careful getting in and out of cars. A bit too quick and you'll give the world an eyeful.

◆ If you choose to go commando, don't get drunk and enter the pub's limbo competition.

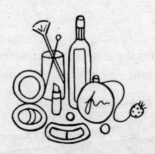

- If you have highlighted hair, beware of strobe lights. You may know the latest dance move but your hair will be green which won't help your cause.

- Don't allow a pissed bloke to light a cigarette for you – he could set fire to your eyebrows and they take a while to grow back. There is certainly no such thing as barefaced chic.

- If you're going out straight from work, keep a stash of emergency fresheners in a desk drawer. A hairbrush, small selection of make-up and a bottle of scent should do it.

- Avoid eating garlic, chilli sauce, spinach or curry if you're planning on a snog.

- Don't fart during your chat-up routine – silent can be deadly.

- If you're having a bad hair day, get over it. Tie it up, make the most of bandanna fashion or plait it. Do not take the baseball-cap option.

- Do not get a radical new haircut or colour the day of a big date – you've got enough to be nervous about. Book an appointment at least two days before. Although, getting a professional blow-dry is an instant beautifier and risk-free.

- Don't overdo the perfume, you'll knock him out at 20 paces and he'll think you're disguising a BO problem.

- To show you're interested, play with your hair, lick your lips, mimic his body position and keep eye contact. If he does the same, you're in there, girl.

- If he appears fidgety and can't keep still he's either married or finds you boring.

- Don't do comical regional accents until you know him better – you don't know who you could be offending. Likewise, racist, homophobic and sexist comments are always inappropriate but unforgivable when you're getting to know someone.

◆ Everyone has to play games but be as honest and upfront as you can with your body language and even if you're playing hard to get, he'll know to take your phone number.

◆ Items of clothing that ALL men find off-putting (leave them for girls' nights) are grey tights, shell suits, boy band T-shirts, cardigans, and sloppy sweatshirts.

◆ Dungarees and cropped hair suggests lesbian. If you have adopted this style and are having trouble pulling, consult a fashion adviser.

◆ Keep jewellery to a minimum – he'll be scared to take you for a boogie on the dance floor in case you jingle too much, and don't wear rings on your wedding finger (unless you are married, in which case this book doesn't really apply).

Chapter Six

Spotting a winner

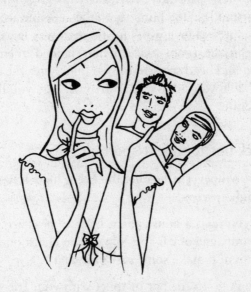

ENOUGH ABOUT YOU, let's get down to him. There's no point looking hot to trot if you're staying in all the time. You've got to get moving – start sharking, pulling, charming and bewitching. Now's the time to get out there and flirt till it hurts. You can't win the raffle unless you buy a ticket...

Detecting the talent

When you first arrive in a bar, club, or party, don't scan the room with wide eyes and your tongue hanging out. A modern girl knows how to be subtle. Prince Charming could be nibbling at the prawn vol-au-vents on the dance floor but you've got all the time in the world to find him. So try to stay cool. Catch up with your friends. Go to the bar and get a round in. Go to the loo and check your lip-gloss. These few natural activities will give you plenty of opportunities to hunt out the eligible men casually. Whoever said love waits for no man was lying. If you rush in, scan the room like a newly landed alien with X-ray vision and head straight for the hunk with the six-pack, not only will you annoy your friends, but you'll look really desperate.

Quick tips for talent-spotting

◆ Ask whoever is hosting the event for a low-down on the singles present.

◆ If you're at a house party, offer to pass around a tray of champagne or canapés so you can check out the wedding rings and make some easy chit-chat.

◆ Don't go to the bar or toilet with your friends. You'll be too busy gossiping to look, and interested males won't be so tempted to smile or make eye contact if you're nattering nineteen to the dozen with a mate.

◆ Set yourself some guidelines to allow quick elimination: if you're only interested in men over 6 ft, don't allow your eye to wander towards dwarves.

◆ Don't get too pissed too early, or forget your contact lenses or glasses if you're shortsighted. You don't want to waste your time flirting with a mongoose or miss opportunities that may lie across the room.

Making a connection

You've seen him, he's gorgeous, you've stopped dribbling and can finally stand up straight without your knees knocking together. How can you get his attention? Well, don't wave manically and yell 'cooeee' across the crowd. And certainly don't moonwalk to the dance area and let loose a Bee Gees-style pointing extravaganza. You can be much more casual. Men aren't as stupid as we think. Well, when there's a snog in it, they're not.

SASHA, 28

❝ Sometimes you have to make the first move. I went into a bar one night and saw this nice guy standing at the bar, talking to his friend. I went to buy drinks for my friends and said hello to him, trying to drum up some sort of conversation. He told me that some girls had shafted him and his mate the previous night – they'd spent a fortune on drinks for them and then the girls buggered off. So this sexy guy said I could only talk to them if I bought them both a drink. I think I must have had a few as I agreed and we carried on chatting until he bought me a drink back. Five years and a wedding later we are still together – so it did pay to be confident and not waste too much time. When you see something you like, go for it. ❞

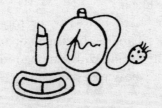

How to bewitch a man without opening your mouth?

Use positive body language (see chapter 5) – especially work those eyes. Let him catch you looking at him, hold his gaze for three seconds (no longer, he'll think you're a stalker) and smile a little – not a lot, toothy grins are not acceptable at this stage. If you're on a dance floor, give it some welly. Be sexy – but not obviously for his benefit (he might try and slip a banknote in your bra). Slow down the moves, unless it is impossible. You'll look ridiculous bumping and grinding to 'The Locomotion'. Use your drink to flirt: suck that straw, nibble that cherry… slip that umbrella behind your ear and shout: 'Arrriibbbbba!' Only joking about the umbrella but the rest can be quite sexy.

He'll be able to tell you're interested (without you dribbling on the floor) if…

- you fidget with your clothing (men think you're inviting them to stare);

- you raise your eyebrows – he'll think this is very naughty;

- you mimic his actions (copying is the sincerest form of flattery);

- you touch your lips, neck and thighs – it will remind him of sex;

- you keep crossing and uncrossing your legs. Do this slowly and he'll be driven wild with expectation but to bystanders, you're just waiting at the bar for a drink – very subtle, we like it.

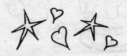

> **NB Drinks say a lot about a girl from a distance.** Avoid rounds of tequila with salt and lemon, or swilling and downing yards of ale or Bloody Marys – for charismatic cocktails stick to Strawberry Daiquiris, Caipirinhas and Blueberry Martinis. Piña Coladas say Essex. A girl will always seem cool asking for a G 'n' T, a vodka tonic or a rum and Coke. Beer says bloke. White-wine spritzers say horsy toff. Whisky says old-timer. Soft drinks say boring or recovering alcoholic. Alcopops say: 'Wahoo, we're on a hen night'. Drink with caution and never drink and drive.

Words of love

You've seductively slurped and sashayed your way through the early evening and now is the time to get the conversation going. If you've been working it properly, you won't have to say or do a thing. He'll be straight over on the third smile. When he does approach you, let's hope he lives up to expectations. He should not mention sex, politics, religion, his mother or farting in the first five minutes. He should openly flirt with you, so you both know where you stand, but he shouldn't be overly sexual.

25 popular pick-up lines

If you hear these, girls, turn on your heel and run... they're out there and they're working on the undereducated modern girl.

1. I wish you were a door so I could slam you all day.

2. Nice legs... what time do they open?

3. Do you work for the post office? I thought I saw you checking out my package.

4. You've got 206 bones in your body. Want one more?

5. Can I buy you a drink or do you just want the money?

6. I may not be the best-looking guy in here, but I'm the only one talking to you.

7. I'm a birdwatcher and I'm looking for a Big-Breasted Bed Thrasher. Have you seen one?

8. I'm fighting the urge to make you the happiest woman on earth tonight.

9. Wanna play army? I'll lie down and you can blow the hell outta me.

10. I wish you were a Pony Carousel, so I could ride you all day long for 20 pence.

11. Oh, I'm sorry, I thought that was a Braille name tag.

12. I'd really like to see how you look when I'm naked.

13. Is that a ladder in your stockings or the stairway to heaven?

14. You must be the limp doctor because I've got a stiffy.

15. Are those real?

16. I'd walk a million miles for one of your smiles, and even farther for that thing you do with your tongue.

17. If it's true that we are what we eat, then I could be you by morning.

18. (Looking at his crotch) Well, it's not just going to suck itself.

19. You. Me. Whipped cream. Handcuffs. Any questions?

20. Fuck me if I'm wrong, but is your name Helga Titsbottom?

21. Wanna come over for some pizza and sex? No? Why? Don't you like pizza?

22. Do you sleep on your stomach? Can I?

23. Do you wash your pants in Windolene? Because I can see myself in them.

24. I lost my puppy. Can you help me find him? I think he went into this cheap motel room.

25. (Lick finger and wipe on her shirt) Let's get you out of these wet clothes.

These ridiculously popular chat-up lines are not acceptable unless you have a very laddish sense of humour and a relaxed attitude to predatory chit-chat. I would seriously advise a swift smile and an emergency dash to the loo if your dream mate begins to use these as part of his pulling technique.

A decent man will strike up a conversation by asking you about yourself, offering to buy you a drink in the first fifteen minutes and keeping the tone light. No mention should be made of dead relatives or criminal records before he's told you what he's doing at that particular venue tonight.

LISA, 30

❝ I was so fed up with the standard of men in this bar. They'd all swan over, stare at my tits and ask me what I did for a living. Then they'd ask me again because they were obviously so busy looking at my chest, they weren't listening the first time. Then this really cute-looking man, who had been observing from a distance, smiled over at me and handed me a bottle of beer. He asked me if I was okay and shuffled along to hear my answer. He said he'd noticed me as soon as I walked in and hadn't been able to take his eyes off me all night. We spent the rest of the evening laughing, dancing and listening to each other's stories. The word to describe our conversation was balanced. We weren't too flirty, or personal, or competitive. We felt friendly from the start and it was the sexiest thing in the world. And he didn't so much as glance at my boobs – or if he did, he was too polite to be unsubtle about it. ❞

Tuning your in-built lie detector

Lots of men are skilled in the art of saying exactly what women want to hear. Like car salesmen, they know how to get a buyer for a clapped-out death machine. I'm not saying you should go into every conversation you might have with a potential date listening out for key words and twitching with suspicion but do pick up on his general manner. Is he overselling himself? If he is, ask yourself why he feels the need to persuade you that he's a good guy. Does he change his opinion on things when you show a preference? If so, he's just saying what you want to hear. Or what he thinks you want to hear. If he quotes lines from films he's probably a bit of a tosser (he must sit in front of the mirror reciting them). He may come out with blatant untruths about life in general thinking you won't know better than him... you can get rid of this sexist pig instantly.

If it's left to you to start conversation...

Make it look like a casual question – then he'll have to respond. You'll both know the game you're playing but it will be easier to start communication. Use the classics:

◆ Do you have a light?

◆ Do you know where the loos are?

◆ Do you have a taxi firm's phone number?

◆ Have I seen you before?

◆ My friend fancies your friend (only stitch your mate up if he's amazing)

◆ Did I leave my drink over here?

◆ Can you believe the slow service in here tonight?

◆ Does the DJ take requests?

◆ Do you have change for the cloakroom, phone etc?

If you're feeling brave and sexy, here are some lines the guys go wild for:

◆ Is my shirt see-through?

◆ I've just been for a manicure; can you get the keys out of my back pocket?

◆ Can you settle a debate: my friend thinks boxers, I think commando?

- Leaving now? Too bad, I was just about to hit on you.

- I always sleep naked – and you?

- Here's my mobile. Tell your flatmate you won't be home tonight.

- This shirt is itchy; I wish I could take it off.

- Hi. I'm conducting a sex survey with my friends and…

- I've had a tough day. I need to de-stress. Any ideas?

- Do you like this scent? (Offer your neck.)

If you can't get a free-flowing chat going (unless it's because the sexual chemistry is so strong you haven't come up for air since he introduced himself), something's wrong. As a modern girl, you'll need to be holding up your end of the bargain: keeping eye contact, listening intently, asking leading questions and talking openly about yourself in a friendly manner. If he's not having any of it, ditch him. If he can't keep his side of the social bargain, he's dumb, disinterested or drunk.

> **NB Don't flog a dead horse.** Unless of course he's a supermodel, in which case buy him a drink and snog his socks off, then say your goodbyes and put it all down to experience. Every girl should snog an outrageously handsome man by the time she's 40, even if he's as dull as ditch-water.

Pull the other one

Even if your eye was initially drawn to Bloke Number One, if, after a bit of banter and a few drinks at the bar, you realise you may have more in common with Bloke Number Two, the friend who came over for moral support, no worries. Ditch the dog and get with the dude. You're not committed to the guy because he bought you a white wine spritzer. The friend may not be interested in you of course – he might not trust you batting your eyelids at him when you were doing it to his buddy an hour ago. Keep it friendly with both of them, just switch your focus to the friend, ask him more direct questions and do a few subtle arm-touches etc. Don't pounce on him when his mate goes to the loo. And don't slag off his mate when you're left alone. That's not big or clever.

NB Don't come on to a mate's bloke. It is never acceptable for a modern girl to come on to a mate's bloke. Even if she's done no more than wink at him during the slow songs, she's nabbed him. There's nothing worse than a girl who lacks imagination and has to wait for a man to be 'accepted' before she finds him attractive. If you suspect a mate is trying to flirt with a bloke she knows you fancy, give her what for. I'm not suggesting hair-pulling at dawn, but let her know her behaviour upsets you.

The 30-minute checklist

After 30 minutes of light-hearted banter, or lusty lip-licking (depending on the amount of sexual chemistry), you should have been able to detect a few things:

◆ Is he single?

◆ Is he more interested in himself than you?

◆ Is he able to hold a conversation?

◆ Is he tight? (If he hasn't offered you a drink, he is.)

◆ Does he have a weak bladder? (Has he been to the loo?)

◆ Does he have good dress sense?

◆ Does he suffer from halitosis, dandruff or body odour?

◆ Does he have shiny shoes (mums find this important)?

If the answers to the above suit you, yippee! You can continue to the next stage... no, not making him fall in love with you. All you need to achieve tonight is getting him to take your phone number, email or arrange a date for a few days' time. You make him fall in love with you then.

How to swap details?

Okay, don't scrawl it over his forehead in lipstick. He might think of you as soon as he wakes up and looks in the mirror the following morning but that won't be a good thing if he's got a hangover. You can be subtler. If you work near each other, suggest a lunch date and give him your professional email in a 'Have you tried the new Italian opposite my office?' line. If the conversation turns to film, music or theatre, find a mutual must-see (even if you have to exaggerate your interest for the sake of a date) and ask him if he wants to go. If you fancy being a straightforward seductress, unclip your handbag and while you're sexily reapplying your lip-gloss, take out a beautifully designed business card and say: 'You'll be wanting this. It's been great talking to you. I should go now,' and make an elegant exit. He'll be gagging for it (even if he wasn't before) – no man can resist a slick application of lip-gloss.

In theory, he should see a good thing when it's standing in front of him and will ask for your number before you have to worry. If he does, be calm. Look pleased but be cool. No gushing or whooping. A simple: 'Of course, it would be nice to hook up' will suffice. Think in advance what details you're prepared to give out up front. Dithering will make you look like you've never been asked out on a date before. Email is a less scary option for both of you – that first phone call can be panic-attack inducing. But if he's a man he can take the pressure, so do what you feel most comfortable with. Mobile numbers are good because you can check who's calling you before you answer – also good if in the cold light of day you realise he was more flunky than hunky. If he rings on a home or work number and you've changed your mind, feign ignorance. A few: 'No sorry, who?' lines and he'll get the hint. Cruel but quick.

> **NB It's your prerogative.** If you bump into someone you refused to date, ignore him if at all possible. If he makes eyes across the dance floor, smile and then ignore him. If he has the guts to approach you, be pleasant. A modern girl never forgets her manners. But don't feel bad and agree to a date, or be persuaded into a snog, or even giving an explanation for your off-hand behaviour. It's your prerogative to date who you want to date and everyone's allowed to change his or her mind.

If he's nervous and doesn't actually get around to taking your number after he's asked you out, remind him. If he gives you his number, don't panic. It's a compliment. He likes you a lot and, if anything, is worried you're out of his league. He wants to see you again but he's left the ball in your court.

If you're both a little shy (how old-fashioned of you!) and don't swap numbers, get the low-down on his social calendar. Plug him for info on where he drinks, eats, goes to the gym. Yes, ask the dreaded question: 'Do you come here often?' It means you can bump into him again in less-suspicious surroundings than his gym on the other side of town. When you get the info, I don't suggest that you start stalking in nutty-bird mode – certainly no lurking around the condom counter at his nearest chemist. But if you happen to run into each other again a few weeks later in a club – fabulous. Everything happens for a reason.

NB It's all in a name. Remember all you need is a surname to get more info on a new love interest. The Internet is wonderful for finding out info without him ever knowing. It can be as personal as school info, or as incongruous as to what his surname means. Very good for passing rainy lunch hours at work.

Even though he might be too shy to say it, he likes you if...

◆ his feet point towards you;

◆ he's touching his face as he looks at you;

◆ he's pointing to his willy – literally, he wants to remind you it's there. I don't mean a big Tony Manero-style dance move, just hands on waist, fingers pointing downwards;

◆ he glances at your mouth on more than one occasion;

◆ he's practically pinned you up against the wall while chatting;

◆ he pulls his socks up (sign of peacock-type grooming).

The rejection section

You may look like a million dollars, sound as witty as Jennifer Aniston in a good episode of *Friends* and dance like a sassy sex queen with Britney's shoes on, but if he doesn't see it, you've lost out. As George Michael said, it is difficult to make someone love you if you don't. Sad but true, sexual chemistry can sometimes be a one-way thing. You can persevere, but men normally decide if they fancy someone in the first minute. They weigh up face, body, hair, attitude and voice and decide if it's a package they want delivered pretty sharpish.

You can tell he's not interested if...

♦ he encourages his friends to stick by his side;

♦ he doesn't offer to buy you a drink;

♦ he doesn't look you in the eye;

♦ not only does he not ask about you, he doesn't even bother to talk about himself... and he yawns;

♦ he stands with his arms crossed and looks around the room for something more interesting;

♦ he takes or makes phone calls and looks at his watch;

♦ he gets your name wrong (perhaps deliberately).

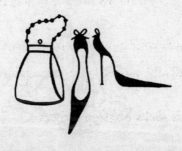

If the loser does any of the above, console yourself with the fact he must be blind, stupid or probably taken already. Besides you've got it all – never think otherwise. If you get the feeling you are being discarded, scarper first. Don't hang on hoping he'll change his mind. Go back to your friends, dance, drink and be merry. Start sharking again if you've got some time left. Do not stare at him wistfully or bore your friends with future-children fantasies. It ain't gonna happen. Be dignified and don't spend another second thinking about what might have been.

Ending the perfect evening

We all moan about the game playing but if we're honest, this can be the most fun stage of the dating process. You've spotted him; he's spotted you. You've danced, flirted, drunk, and giggled a little too much. And you've swapped numbers at the end of it. You've bumped and grinded to the slow songs at the end (and even managed to snog your way through the extended remix of Spandau Ballet's 'True'). Agreed, there's still a lot of uncertainty – he may not call, he may turn out to be a loser, you may marry him, have three children and then discover he's a transvestite. Nothing in love is cut and dried. Nothing. So enjoy the adrenalin and endorphins you get from this initial contact. You came, you saw, you conquered.

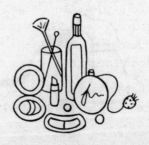

Secrets of Success

◆ Make sure you've read all previous chapters. Preparation is everything.

◆ Do not make Benny Hill-style facial expressions at the man of your dreams. Gurning is not a good look. He'll think you're having a panic attack rather than flirting.

◆ Never under any circumstance fight with another girl in public because of a man. His ego will be boosted to the point where he won't want either of you, and you'll get bruised and possibly fall over.

◆ If you strike up a chat and he says he hates smoking, do not strike a match. This is your cue to hide your cigarettes if you like him.

◆ Don't chew gum. You'll look like a grazing cow.

◆ Think about investing in one of those new tiny digital cameras – then, on the pretext of capturing the memorable night, reel off a few shots of your target. End result – you'll be able to conduct an email post-mortem with your mates the next day.

◆ Do not try to impress him with the formation dancing you and your chums learnt last week in keep fit.

◆ Pick a venue full of available men for your sharking expedition. Avoid gay bars, parish quiz evenings, boutique openings, Westlife concerts... and avoid going out Sunday, Monday and Tuesday nights. Single people are exhausted after their weekend pursuits.

◆ Make sure you have enough cash to buy drinks and get a taxi if you stay longer than you should and miss the last bus, or train.

- Avoid regressing to an eleven-year-old. The pack mentality of some girls out on the pull – guffawing loudly and limboing on the bar – is a turn-off to most men. Have fun with your mates but when he makes a move, move away so you can concentrate without your friends pinching your arse and whispering 'wa-hey' in your ear.

- If you feel it's important to get an abridged relationship history, do so with subtlety. Ask roundabout questions like does he live on his own? How long for? Mention your last ex and gauge how he responds. However, the ex-files can be left until a few dates in to a relationship (except if there are children involved).

- Eliminate swiftly. Don't waste your time on someone you know isn't right for you. It sounds a bit abrupt but you can't persuade yourself to fancy someone. It's better to have a good night out with the girls than talk to someone you'll never see again.

- Don't be put off if he dances badly. Most men do.

- Brief your friends not to tell any embarrassing stories about you.

- Brief your friends to rescue you from a dodgy bloke – use a certain look (a wink, a scratch) or a noise (a cough) to make them intervene. Obviously tell them the code before you go out or you could be coughing all night to no avail.

- Watch out if he doesn't disagree with you once in your conversation. He's trying too hard and is the kind of guy to buy you stuffed animals.

- If you are lonely or insecure, you may fall for the wrong kind of guy. Remember at all times you are the fabulous one.

◆ Women are drawn to bastards. Who knows why? All you'll get from them is a broken heart, sleepless nights and a self-esteem crisis. By the time you're 30 you should have learnt this. Bastards aren't more exciting. They're just immature. Good men aren't dull and they are good in bed. They are just comfortable enough with themselves not to have to treat girls badly to make themselves feel important.

◆ Flirting is fabulous. Flirting makes you feel sexy. Even if the talent has hit an all-time low on a certain night, practise for the future with a little light-hearted minxing. Do flirt with women too.

◆ Never make eyes at a man who is talking to another woman. That's just rude.

◆ Don't use your hands too much when you're trying to lure Mr Perfect into your web. A playful punch on the arm is fine; grabbing his arse is not.

◆ If a nice-guy-but-no-way asks for your phone number and you're never going to see him again, you are allowed to tell a white lie and say you are seeing someone to protect his feelings. Even add in a line like: 'Otherwise, I'd love to...' Never say that you are a lesbian – this can make them want you even more...

◆ A modern girl can ask a man out if they've been chatting all evening. Some men even find it sexy and bold. Just remember, if you asked him, you may have to pay for dinner – but who cares if he's gorgeous?

◆ Have fun.

Chapter Seven

Courtship clues

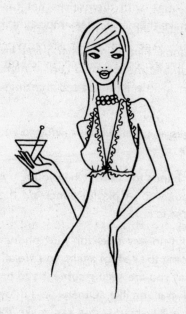

Y OU MET HIM, you liked him... and you hope he's
going to say yes when you call him for a drink – or
even better, that your answering machine is already
blinking away with the news of a message from lover boy.
But what did you really get to know about him during the
course of the evening when – let's face it – you could have
both had a little too much to drink? It could have been
quite dark, and you suffer from new-man amnesia (you
think he said witty, intelligent things and he had nice eyes
but you can't be sure now).

Identikit man

Quickly! Before you forget everything about this new man, make a note of his characteristics and think about whether you can live with them. This means relying on stereotypes and isn't entirely politically correct but, at this very early stage in the dating game, any piece of info you can deduce from him is good. And remember, stereotypes exist for a reason, i.e. they are generally, loosely based on the truth. So get analysing.

Your mother warned you...

There are certain men who show up in every example of romantic literature and costume drama. This is because so many women can relate to them. All 'obvious' men (see below) have their pros and cons – can you balance them?

The toy boy

If you can get over the initial embarrassment and outrage at the age difference from those around you, this could be a very fulfilling relationship. It is a celebrated fact that women reach their sexual peak in their 40s, while men flourish in their early 20s, so keep the relationship in the bedroom and you'll have lots of fun. Leave your sin den and things may get tricky. Different tastes in music, film, style etc may seem shallow but can cause arguments. His friends will make you feel old and he may expect you to go shopping with his mother. He may also be a little commitment-shy.

The sugar daddy

The confidence, wealth and contacts that come with an older man can seem very attractive. He's been around the block and knows how to treat a lady... but unfortunately he also knows how he likes to be treated. He may be a bit stuck in his ways and, let's say it, a little chauvinistic. I'm not saying he'll chain you to the sink, and let you off your lead once a week to visit his boudoir, but he may have a few issues with the lifestyle choices of the modern girl. He's more rheumatic than romantic.

The married man

To start with, a married man may be the answer to your 'sex and dinner but no fuss' fantasy. And of course, when you hit 35 most good men seem to be hitched already and you need to plough this field for a decent conversation. And of course, some men don't tell you they're married until you're loved up. An affair may seem glamorous to start with but it soon descends into guilt, shame and ultimately him deciding to stay with his wife. So moral standpoint aside, think about your own heart and self-respect before you become his bit on the side.

The charmer

He's so smooth he has trouble sitting upright on a leather sofa. This guy oozes charm, one-liners and compliments. Some of your friends see through this straight away but you're enjoying the attention. He makes you feel like the sexiest woman alive so enjoy it – but don't trust him or get used to having him around. This Casanova is also a chronic cheat. He loves women so much, as he keeps telling you, that one just isn't enough (modern girls should read between the lines, i.e. he doesn't love women at all, he loves his dick).

The boy-next-door

Not literally of course but you know what I mean. The lad you've known for years. You share friends, history, and chewing gum. Your mother thinks he's great and your father soon relies on him for trips to the DIY centre. Herein lies the rub. The fact he's Mr Popular with everyone else makes him a bit of a lick-arse in your eyes. The more your mum coos, the more you want to chuck. If this relationship has a chance, keep him away from your relatives for a while so you can decide if he's a keeper – before they do.

The commitment-phobe

At first you think his aloofness is alluring. You have fun when you are together, the sex is great and he pays for his share of drinks but he's still playing hard to get. Soon, what once seemed alluring turns annoying. He won't introduce you to his friends or family, he never returns your calls, and he shirks out of nights in front of the telly *chez vous*. He doesn't handle confrontation well and would rather avoid you than answer any grown-up questions. He's not ready for a sophisticated modern girl yet. If he's lucky, you'll still be around in a few years when he's realised what he had.

The bisexual

Why limit yourself to one gender? Love should be for all. Well, that's what he's tried to tell you anyway and at first you're convinced. Sexual attraction is about souls, not whether someone has boobs or a willy – how completely shallow were you before? Come on! Is this freedom of expression – yes – but is it fair to you – no! This is a lifestyle choice and if you haven't chosen it, it's difficult. You may think your man getting cosy with Alan from the office wouldn't be as bad as if he'd picked Tina but that's not the case. If he's with you, it should be 100%. If he's still insisting on drinking from both cups, turn off your Soda Stream.

Mr Trauma

This guy has had it tough. His parents were horrible to him; he was picked on at school, his ex-wife cheated on him... he needs to be looked after. Step in 'super modern girl'. You can save him with your honesty, good heart and healing hands. He makes you feel like you have an aim, a project. It's only a few months into his moaning you start to understand why the others treated him badly – he's a pain. He never takes responsibility for his own life and is dependent on self-help books. Ditch him before he drags you down with him. It's better to be the bitch that broke his heart.

Occupational hazards

A sad but true state of affairs in modern life is that your job defines you... we all know the dinner-party dilemma – can you wait more than two minutes to ask the person next to you what they do for a living? Probably not. Someone's choice of career says more about them than how they did at school – it allows an instant insight into their income, lifestyle, social circle, and ambition – and of course future prospects... all things a prospective date needs to know. So, confronting sweeping generalisations in the face, here is a mini guide to handling all types of job while you're on the job.

Accountants

Perhaps they have an unfair reputation as penny-pinching bores – but hey, where there's smoke there's usually fire. Unfortunately for an accountant's date the only flames of passion she'll ignite are when she's discussing her tax returns over an expenses-reclaimable dinner. There are pros though of course: he's not a gambler, your parents will approve and you'll never have to grimace in confusion at your bank statements again. Just avoid his office parties like the plague.

Rock star

Rock, pop, soul and rap... any kind of musician is likely to be more obsessed with his instrument (and I'm not talking about the one he slings over his shoulder after a gig – unless you're a very lucky girl) than you. To stand up on stage you have to have a fairly huge ego and this doesn't do much for his caring and sensitive side, unless he's a Bob Dylan type.

Model

The beautiful guy is good at two-way relationships – between himself and the mirror. Come on girls, admit it – you may think dating a model is a good idea, for about two weeks. You soon realise that even an inbox full of bitter emails from friends can't compensate for the fact he only ever orders a salad when you go out for dinner. And the trouble with looking so good – for men and women – is that they don't have to work on the rest of it as much.

Bankers

Bankers, traders, brokers et al have a reputation for being wide boys with much wallet power but little brainpower. And of course the side effect of having such fast-paced, high-octane work lives is that they need extra stimulus to keep them social – and I don't mean an in-depth conversation about the future of British theatre. Always good for champers and share tips though.

Marketing and PR

These guys can be a little bitter because no one really knows what they do… and then when they work it out, they think it sounds like a bit of a girl's job. And it may be – it involves lots of smarming, schmoozing, wining and dining, getting overexcited about shopping and wearing designer clothes. These guys could sell Eskimos a fridge so be sure you see through the sales speak when they're persuading you out on a second date.

Footballers

Yes, they're fit, rich, and popular with everyone in the pub and look good in a pair of shorts. But are you really happy to be known as a footballer's wife? You'd soon be defined as the stereotypical peroxide bimbo with no brains, and if you are, you might want to at least pretend to be a little more enigmatic. And all that washing of dirty kits before he hits the big time, public brawls, and rude chanting could drive you mad.

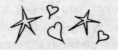

Civil servants

These guys can be jobsworths. Before you know it you'll be told you shouldn't wear blue and black together, you shouldn't really have a snack before dinner, that drinking Blue Nun really isn't acceptable anymore. These boys are sticklers for rules, so if you get off on the dominant, sadomasochist thing, then you're sorted. If you're looking for freedom, excitement and fly-by-the-seat-of-your-pants decisions, don't go there.

Artists

For artist also read moody. Yes, they're creative, deep and romantic but they're also potentially self-obsessed, depressive and serious. Good for a fling – you could have a poem or sculpture dedicated to you and, as we saw in *Ghost,* a lot of fun can be had with clay. Just be prepared for the mood swings when the rest of the world doesn't think their work is as earth-shatteringly amazing as you do.

Handymen and builders

If you can put up with them leering (these are the only occupation who actively live up to their stereotype) at poor office workers as they make their way to work, go for it. The benefits of having a man around the house who can plaster, paint, mend and fix are endless – even if you do have to get an eyeful of his denim-clad buttock crevice while he's doing it.

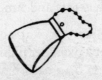

Lawyers

They'd sooner argue than look at you. They love a good fight, this bunch, and oh yes, they've always got to be right. They're armed with facts, figures and an encyclopaedic knowledge of misdemeanours. Good for advice and impressing the family; just make sure you're strong enough to put up with the in-depth debates you'll be forced to have over breakfast every morning.

Dating a celebrity

Women's magazines insist that everyone should sleep with a star by the time they are 25. To be honest, you'd probably have to achieve this aim by the time you're 30 – or even 20 – because most male celebs like them young, taut and very, very thin. If you do want to 'do' a star bear the following in mind.

Don't be too fussy

Obviously there aren't enough A-listers like Brad Pitt and George Clooney to go round; so many modern girls looking for a bit of the limelight will have to look lower down the celebrity scale. Luckily, thanks to satellite television, reality game shows and an influx of celebrity magazines out there, there's plenty to choose from. On a sliding scale:

- ◆ A-list dates: American actors and British rock stars.

- ◆ B-list dates: British actors and American rock stars.

- ◆ C-list dates: Soap stars – okay so they're not the best-looking bunch but your grandma will approve and millions watch them on a daily basis.

- D-list dates: Sportsmen, particularly footballers, are very rich and stupid enough not to know how quickly you're spending it.

- E-list dates: Social climbers – they normally stick to models, but your eyes could meet over a racetrack one day (good for getting into bars).

- F-list dates: Television presenters are universally acknowledged as being sunny, bright and generally good with animals and children.

- Z-list dates: Has-beens, i.e. anyone who looks familiar but you can't quite place the face or name. Don't knock them; they will still get tickets to restaurant openings so they have their uses.

Do make them feel special

You'd assume paying people to lick their arse all day long would get their need for being worshipped out of the way, but no – they want it 24/7. If you went down on your knees and kissed their shoes, stars would think you were just giving them their deserved respect. You see, they thrive on feeling special, being the best and telling everyone else what to do. If you want to be with them, you'll have to get in line with the hired help and start singing their praises.

Don't try to overshadow them

Under no circumstances should you wear a more expensive, revealing, or sexy outfit when in a place you could be spotted. You should not have a nicer car, better hair or whiter teeth. You must maintain a certain level of grooming if you want to be on their arm, but do not – for one minute – think you can compete.

Do keep it a secret

Whatever you do, don't ring up the tabloids and offer to strip down to your red, lacy negligee and reveal all about his massive hot tub and small penis... not until he's dumped you for a page three girl anyway (then get yourself an agent and sell your story to the highest bidder).

Don't beat up his fans

Yes, they are annoying and tend to scream or cry all the time but they are the paying public. If it weren't for these losers (you're with him after all, not them), you wouldn't be going to Mauritius on holiday this year. So be gracious and take a back seat. Don't flaunt your happiness in their faces until you've got a rock on your finger. Then they'll have to lump it.

Do get chummy with his staff

If you don't get in quick with his road, tour, or personal manager or his press people, you'll be cut out of his schedule and, thus, out of his life. If his bodyguards normally fix him up with groupies backstage, you need to make sure you're there. Buying them doughnuts and coffee usually does the trick.

Don't stress out if you're ignored

Honey, you chose to date a celebrity. It can be great: the money, the travel, the adoration... but it can be cold out in his shadow. Focus on the good things – and take solace in the fact that relationships in the spotlight don't usually last long. So you'll be back with an accountant who adores you before you know it.

Get the scope from his horoscope

If love is written in the stars, make sure you're picking up the right signs. You can tell a lot about a man by his horoscope – good and bad, here are the characteristics to look out for.

Capricorn (December 22–January 20)

What a lovely man! Capricorns are known for their good humour, kindness and patience. They make everyone feel content... until life does them wrong. Then they can fall quickly into pessimism and begrudge people with more than them. Appeal to their disciplined side and you can keep them on a steady path.

Aquarius (January 21–February 19)

What a fun one the Aquarian is... friendly, original and inventive – you'll get a lot from talking to him alone. He's very intelligent. Only problem is he knows it and can be a little contrary, perverse and detached if he wants to win an argument. Stick up for yourself or you'll be swallowed while your friends all tell you how lucky you are for having such a livewire as a date.

Pisces (February 20–March 20)

There's something fishy going on with this guy... you'll never know where you stand with him. One minute he's being sensitive to your needs, the next he's being secretive and shutting you out. He is kind – don't get me wrong – but he's weak-willed and escapist, which can make him a bit unreliable.

Aries (March 21–April 20)

He's not nicknamed the ram for nothing – this guy is adventurous and energetic (in and out of bed) and enthusiastic and confident enough to make sure you have a good time too. The problem is perhaps he's a bit too impulsive and you might find his daredevil side difficult to control. His quick temper could annoy you as well.

Taurus (April 21–May 21)

This guy is warm-hearted and loving, persistent and determined. He's passionate about life and for a while will be passionate about you. Be careful however. His passion can quickly turn into jealousy and possessiveness and he could resent your freedom or success. The bull sign highlights his stubbornness and self-indulgence.

Gemini (May 22–June 21)

Expect to be dating two men – a good twin and an evil twin. When he's happy, expect to be with a witty, youthful and lively chap. When he's not, expect him to be superficial, nervous and cunning. Make sure you can handle the rough with the smooth or he'll give you a nervous breakdown.

Cancer (June 22–July 23)

This is a crab of the hermit variety. All a Cancer man wants is stability, a proper home and a loving partner (a wife preferably). If you're looking to settle down, hunt out this protective and loving type. If you're not, avoid him like the plague: he can be clingy, emotional and moody if you don't return his feelings.

Leo (July 24–August 23)

Generous and warm-hearted, creative and enthusiastic. Leo man offers the most fun you can have with someone – when he's the centre of attention. If you challenge his sovereignty, he can get pompous, bossy and patronising. To win the heart of this one, treat him like a king and you can be his much-loved queen (with less power than him).

Virgo (August 24–September 23)

This sign is known as the virgin because its birthday boys are modest, shy and intelligent. They want everything to be simple and their relationships to be straight down the line. This is great if you're a clean-cut kind of girl. If you're not he might worry, fuss over you and be a little over-critical. Can you date a perfectionist?

Libra (September 24–October 23)

His balanced attitude to life makes this guy diplomatic, easy-going and sociable. He likes everyone to get on, and that includes the two of you. If you tip the scales, however, expect him to change his mind about you quite quickly. Librans are gullible and easily influenced, and can be easily swayed against you.

Scorpio (October 24–November 22)

Watch out for the sting in this one's tail! You may be attracted by his powerful, passionate and magnetic personality to start with… but this can soon turn to darker things. Prone to jealousy, obsessiveness and compulsiveness. If you want a dramatic fling, go for a Scorpion. If you want an easy life, don't.

Sagittarius (November 23–December 21)

Can you feel the love in this man? He's a hippy through and through. He'll chill you out and slow you down after a busy day in the office or a fight with your best mate. If you are a high-powered career girl you might find his blindly optimistic and careless attitude to life a little irresponsible… but maybe you should change, not him?

What men really want

It's true, most men wouldn't know their arses from their elbows – let alone know what is right for them in the game of love. But in the interests of equal opportunities, I allowed a few to have their say. Handy hints or what?

> **Alan, 35**
> 'Modern girls either try too hard or don't try at all. Turning up in sloppy jeans with no make-up and unkempt hair is not really trying at all… just stay at home if you're going to be like this. But then again, try too hard and the man will be scared to touch you or panic about what you look like underneath the slap.'

James, 26
'When I meet a girl, I try to work out what animal she reminds me of. If it's one that licks its own arse, I won't be asking her out on a date.'

William, 32
'If I knew where to find single birds, I wouldn't be single. Definitely don't hang out looking desperate in nightclubs would be my advice to single men or women. Meeting people through friends or at sophisticated drink-dos (where you can't get too drunk) are definitely the best. You get introduced to the other singletons but there's no grief if you realise halfway through the conversation that they're awful.'

Jason, 28
'The problem with women is that they're not more like men. Unfortunately it's usually up to us to make the effort – first moves, start up conversations, pinch their bums etc. In an ideal world, women would be blokes with boobs. It's such an eye-opener going to gay bars and watching men flirt with men. No one messes around. Everyone makes an effort. But maybe I should stop hanging around with my gay friends – it could explain why I'm still single?'

Johnny, 31
'My most embarrassing night in recent history was going to a singles party on my own. No one spoke to me – even the barman ignored me for half an hour. I assumed that being a singles' event, everyone would be alone, but massive groups were there and weren't integrating. When I did summon up the courage to speak to anyone, they looked at me like: 'I'm

talking to my friend, what the hell do you want?' After an hour, I walked out of the door backwards, laughing at imaginary jokes I was being told by friends I hadn't made. Once I got out the door, I didn't know whether to laugh or cry. To clear my head, I spent two hours walking home.'

Lee, 29

'I don't think sex on a first date is a bad thing. I don't think it means a girl is easy or cheap, but on the rare occasion when a girl does say no – and means it – it can be quite novel. I think a good fumble and 'everything but' can be almost as good when you first get to know them. It makes the whole thing last a bit longer and I suppose ultimately you do have a bit more respect for her. When you do finally get to sleep with them, you feel like you're not just one of many. As if you mean something special to them.'

Dave, 40

'Nothing upsets me more than hairy armpits. It's not modern – and it certainly doesn't mean women are more liberated – it just looks a bit weird and dirty.'

Lawrence, 26

'What a girl wears is always important on the first few dates, but it's what she says and how she interacts socially that is more important. I like it when a girl acknowledges what I've done for her. In fact, nothing annoys me more than buying a girl dinner and her not saying thank you. I know men are supposed to say she looks lovely, take her coat and open doors for women, but this is the age of equality and it doesn't hurt for the girl to compliment you on your efforts. If a girl automatically assumes you'll pick up the tab for the whole evening without asking, I think she's a bit cheeky.'

Steven, 27
'If only all women could bottle the sex appeal 20% of them have. Some women just look like they love sex, that they would ravish you if they got you within ten metres of their bedroom. All men love this. A woman who is confident with her body (whatever the size or shape) and enjoys herself – especially when she's having sex – is priceless.'

Chapter Eight

First dates

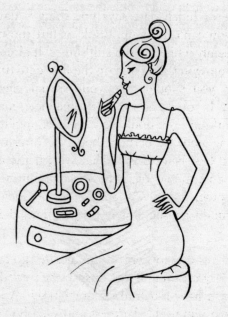

SCARY STUFF. First dates are the worst... well, they're great too because he liked you enough to ask you out, but yikes – what do you do now? In the few hours before you meet him, expect to sweat, pace up and down like a sergeant major and take up smoking again. Or you can take control, stay calm and make yourself look incredible. Modern girls choose the latter option.

Any time, any place, anywhere?

Traditionally, if he asked you out he should pick the venue... but by all means offer suggestions. Here are a few possibilities to discuss:

◆ A coffee or lunch date says one thing – daytime. This means you can't dress up, drink or flirt too much. It's a tad unseemly while the sun still shines. It almost certainly means you won't shag him on the first date (if you do get that far, you should take your sexual chemistry and bottle it). If you do go for a daytime meet, make sure it's not a workday. You don't want to be limited to an hour if it is going well. Or perhaps book the afternoon off but don't tell him beforehand. That way, if the date's lousy you can do a runner, blaming work commitments, and go off shopping; and if it's good you can decadently sit there all afternoon getting slowly tipsy... until the sun starts to fade.

◆ A trip to a show, concert or film dictates no talking. This may be a good thing if you suspect he's good to look at but doesn't have much to say for himself. You can stare lustfully at him in the darkness and snog him on the way home. Some would say you're just delaying the inevitable until the second date but you never know? Maybe Cirque du Soleil will be back in town by then. If you go to the cinema, choose the film carefully. A love story may make him feel uncomfortable and you don't want your make-up to run during the emotional bits. A drama may be too depressing and require too much concentration. A horror film is good if you want an excuse to squeeze his knee, but I would always recommend a comedy. Laughter is a great aphrodisiac.

◆ An exclusive restaurant means he wants to show you off. He thinks you're gorgeous and only worthy of the best. It also means that he's thought long and hard about where to take you for maximum effect. One could argue that he's being flash or trying too hard but always enjoy the experience. Even if he turns out to be a wideboy, you get to sample the lobster and tell your friends about it the following morning.

◆ A suggested trip to his abode for dinner or drinks is to be avoided at all costs. Not only does he think he can have sex without wining or dining you, but you don't know him. He could be an axe murderer... probably not... but a girl should at least observe a gent's table manners before she observes his bedside manner.

◆ Cocktails are always a good option. Of course, you should worry if he orders a girly drink with an umbrella for himself or insists on getting you a Sloe Long Comfortable Screw or a Screaming Orgasm. If you stick with the sensible list and a few olives, you should get nicely acquainted – and if it goes well you have the dinner stage to move on to.

◆ A cheapskate date is never good. If he suggests taking you for a hamburger, suggest otherwise. Not only is it hard to look attractive slurping on a milkshake but you'll also be forced to share your first moments with sulky teens and a children's party. The exception is a well-

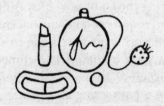

thought-out picnic in a park – by definition this is a cheap date but it is also very romantic... and the true merit depends on what he's got packed in the hamper.

> **NB Choose your food carefully.** There is nothing worse than struggling with a difficult food choice on a first date. Avoid all types of pasta in case of slurping, dribbling, swinging and spilling. For scent reasons give onions, garlic and strong-smelling fish a miss. Don't drink too much coffee – it will make you hyper. And remember that red wine can give you purple teeth (which isn't so much of a problem if you're both drinking it – you can look silly together). Try not to eat finger foods; not only do they leave your hands sticky but you have to shove it all in your gob in one go – where possible try to stick to knife-and-fork food.

As a final point, avoid judging the man too harshly on the setting he's chosen for your meeting. Even the most thoughtful man can get it wrong; it's far more important to judge the intent and how good a time you have in his company. My husband, who normally knows better, thought it would be great to take me to a rainforest-themed restaurant after watching a 3-D film about safaris. Total, total disaster – but his heart was in the right place.

Countdown without collapse

Let's pretend you're meeting him at 8 p.m. Here's how to spend your day:

1. Arrange to see your friends. This will keep you busy and stop too much self-analysis. Go shopping for a first-date outfit or go for a pampering at a spa.

2. Exhaust your nerves at the gym (exercise will also make you feel happier and give you a healthy glow).

3. Don't start getting ready any earlier than 5.30 p.m. You are allowed two glasses of wine for Dutch courage but no more. You'll get red blotches and forget to put any knickers on (which of course you may choose to do, it's a free world). Have a bath or shower, moisturise for soft skin (good for when he gives you a flirty stroke), and apply deodorant (check in the mirror to make sure you haven't got any dodgy white marks).

4. Don't do anything too radical with your hair or make-up in case it traumatises you the whole night long. And don't use too many products, in case he tries to run his fingers through your hair and gets stuck, or removes your tan when he rubs your cheek.

5. Finally, put on your chosen outfit *after* you've applied your make-up, finished cleaning your flat if you've chosen to do so, and polished off any last-minute drinks or snacks.

NB Don't starve yourself before a dinner date. Not least because it's unhealthy but also you don't want to be thinking solely about the food and/or how desperately hungry you are. You should be looking at the guy across the table, not staring wistfully in the direction of the kitchen. Likewise, when you get to the date I don't advise ordering only a lettuce leaf followed by a bowl of water – it sends out one signal: neurotic.

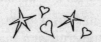

Arriving in style

If you can, get a taxi to the date venue so you arrive clean and unflustered with make-up intact. You want to make a maximum-effect entrance so, rather than arriving early, take a trip to a shop and stock up on chewing gum or something. Anything. Walk through the door of the designated venue five minutes late. Any later would be rude. If he's not there yet, you are more than entitled to set yourself up at the bar with a cocktail and flirt with the bartender. It's your date's fault for being impolite.

But hopefully your date will be there waiting, his eyes will light up when you walk towards him (you won't fall over or run to his arms at great speed) and he'll stand up as you approach. Any decent man on a first date will tell you that you look great (whether he thinks it or not) and pull your chair out for you. This isn't chauvinism; this is chivalry. He'll offer you a drink, both your hearts will be racing but luckily you won't be able to hear each other's. He might be shaking slightly (it's a big deal for him too) and you'll both down the first drink a little too quickly.

How to stay cool when you're on fire

It's important to judge the mood of the evening quite quickly. If you like each other it will be obvious from the start. The fact you've got this far – without the help of beer goggles – is a good sign. If you really like him, look him in the eye and for God's sake, whatever you do, don't tell him! No. Look him in the eye and talk about him, you, the weather. If you tell him you really like him straight away, he'll be tempted to run even if he was thinking the same thing. It's a self-protection reflex all men have. It's much safer to show him you're keen by listening to what he says, asking him questions, dropping hints about films you'd like to see, asking him if he's busy next week... and being irresistible. Under no circumstances ask to meet his mother, demand to know his favourite children's names, or doodle his surname and hearts on a napkin. You have stumbled into psycho-stalker territory.

The first-date interval

A few hours into the date, visit the toilets to powder your nose and take stock. Is this man cool? It's best to weigh things up before you get drunk and it gets late. If you've noticed any of the following, he's probably not the guy for you:

◆ He is rude about all of his ex-girlfriends;

◆ He has a wandering eye;

◆ He complains about the prices at the bar but shows off about his huge salary;

◆ He doesn't make you laugh even once;

◆ He quotes his mother constantly and says you look a bit like her;

◆ He talks into his mobile more than he talks to you;

◆ He's tried to look up your skirt or down your top and calls you bird.

If he hasn't done any of the above, you are indeed a lucky lady. Now what are you doing in the toilets? Get out there and wow him. He sounds pretty hooked already.

Was I mad?

There is always the nightmare scenario that the man who seemed perfect in the smoky nightclub when you'd had a few drinks looks rather different when you meet for coffee in the cold light of day. Even if you don't recall him being shorter than you – with a limp – you made the date so you have to stick with it. Don't let your facial expressions display your disappointment. You don't have to flirt, kiss or promise to see him again but you can't run away if he's being considerate and charming. You won't be such a drunken old soak next time you go out flirting will you?

CLAIRE, 28

❝ Picture the scene - a sunny, spring race meeting at Ascot. In a boozy corporate tent, their eyes lock over the champagne cocktails. A successful, single, client service director (him) meets slightly squiffy, single journalist (me) and they embark on a daylong battle of banter. They arrange a dinner date. Having seen the aforementioned journalist survive several Bridget Jones-style disasters, her erstwhile mates are excited at this new development. 'Well, at least you've spent a day with him, so you know he won't be on his mobile all the time, talk about himself a lot or wear a YELLOW SHIRT,' they squeal, listing their pet hates. That evening, he arrives to pick me up and spends 30 minutes on the phone before barely saying hello. While she polishes off a bottle of wine, he tells her all about his day (for another 30 minutes) before going to 'freshen up' and change into a YELLOW SHIRT. I went on the date but I didn't see him again. ❞

If disaster strikes...

If you're genuinely taken ill, don't try to hide it. Explain you're under the weather and try to get out of there before you start vomiting. That's not a good move on a first date. If he's a gentleman he'll get you safely into a taxi and text or phone you the next day to check you're better. When you next communicate, laugh about your disaster (if you're over the nausea and off the toilet) and tell him that you really enjoyed his company before the bug struck. Suggest you have a second first date and this time you'll behave yourself properly.

If you can't think of anything to talk about – even though you both obviously like each other – go dancing. Let your bodies do the talking. You know you're both keen from the few hours you've spent smiling and staring, so change location, boogie on down and that will give you some new experiences to discuss.

If a family crisis hits while you're out which really needs to be resolved ASAP – that is it's not just a relative being a drama queen – explain quickly and honestly, ask when he's next free and rearrange a date. Apologise wholeheartedly and convince him that you would much rather be talking to him than coping with this unexpected problem. Hopefully he'll admire your kindness and soon come to rely on your good opinions too.

If your dress splits, you spill a drink over yourself, or an alternative fashion faux pas takes place, handle it with good grace and humour. What's done is done. If a damp cloth and a quick blast under the hand-dryer doesn't do the trick, and you're not anywhere near a clothes shop to buy an alternative, sod it. If the date's been going well up to this point, it won't be your clothes he's interested in. Quite the opposite in fact.

If you're running late – and likely to keep him waiting for a while – tell him so he knows he hasn't been stood up. Traffic, weather, a last-minute phone call… all these things can hold up dates. Tardiness will make the other person feel unimportant so if you know you're going to arrive 20 minutes or more later than the designated time, ring him on his mobile or ring the place you're meeting (weigh this one up – it could be embarrassing for him if they loudly announce that you're behind schedule in a packed bar). You should always swap numbers for unexpected occurrences such as these. If you can't contact him and he's still patiently sitting there an hour later, be thankful and apologetic. Don't think for a minute that he's a bit of a loser for waiting. If he's gone, try to understand his plight. Email the next day giving an honest, brief explanation and asking to rearrange.

You're not alone

Under no circumstance is it acceptable for him to bring a friend along with him. If he suggests you go somewhere en masse, suggest he call you again when he can donate a whole evening to you. He'll get the message and dump the friends, or you'll realise you had a lucky escape.

Should you have sex on the first date?

The age-old dilemma never gets any easier to answer. Some people – and women are often more judgemental than men are – believe that a women who has sex on a first date is cheap. This isn't necessarily so, and certainly, if a woman is cheap, so is the man.

A very handsome, popular pop star told me recently that he has two kinds of one-night stands. Firstly, he sleeps with a girl he's not interested in long-term but knows she's up for it, and they both want sex. The second one-night stand is with a girl who he's instantly in love with. Their date goes brilliantly, the sexual chemistry is insurmountable and in the hope that this will become a serious relationship, they fall straight into bed. This guy may have more than his fair share of women throwing themselves at him, but I think most men divide first-date sex into these two categories. Sometimes they just want sex, and sometimes the girls are too amazing to send home.

If a modern girl is hoping for more than a one-night stand from her first date, she needs to learn to read the signs. If you are both drunk, both randy and neither of you can be bothered to get a taxi home, sleep with each other – but don't expect this to be the start of a great love affair. If your first date has been heavenly, if you laugh together and can't stop looking into each other's eyes, and he's a fantastic snogger, you could be having sex with your future husband.

How do you know he has more than coffee on his mind?

If you don't fancy playing the minx and making the first move, you must understand when he's asking you – and when he's not. If he invites you back to his place for coffee, he wants to have sex (or at least something approaching it). As a general rule of thumb a modern girl must understand 'coming back for a drink' means 'sexual shenanigans' and if she *really* fancies an espresso or one last glass of champagne, she should suggest a late-night bar. Likewise, if he suggests a Chinese takeaway back at his when you have to pass three Oriental Chefs to get there, he wants ecstasy with his egg-fried rice. But it is nice of him to offer to feed you afterwards. If you are genuinely hungry for food and food alone, suggest a great restaurant that doesn't do delivery. He'll get the hint.

> **NB Avoid awkward situations.** If he does persuade you to go back to his for 'coffee' – this does not automatically give him a mandate to get frisky without your say-so. Take my advice and avoid getting into this situation if it's unwanted, but if it happens don't feel like you owe him anything you don't feel comfortable doing.

Great expectations

Do not expect the sex to be mind-blowing first time. Every girl wants an orgasm (or more) but realistically you're going to have to wait a little longer for that. If he does give you a mind-blowing head rush, cling on to him... but not in a needy way so he does a runner. Nerves, unfamiliarity and booze can understandably make first-date bedroom gymnastics a little lacklustre. If you really like each other, you could be so nervous the shaking gets too much and he can't keep an erection or lets you know he's excited a little too soon. Take it as a compliment – especially if he admits why. Be aware that if it's a one-night stand session, you won't care about pleasing each other, and this can lead to perfunctory, does-the-job sex.

Rose, 27

❝ I arranged to meet Lee for our first date at a certain bar in London. I used to go there a lot with the guys from work so when I walked in the guy behind the bar said, 'Hi Rose, Bombay Sapphire and tonic?' I was so embarrassed and felt like a right midweek drinker – not the impression I wanted to give Lee at all. Anyway, he was driving so he had 1 pint of beer and 2 lemonades to my 3 double gin and tonics and to say I was then feeling confident would be an understatement – so much so that when he said: 'Where shall we go to get something to eat?' I replied: 'There's a fantastic restaurant called Little Italy right next door to my flat!' How brave was that? So we drove back to my flat, parked up and as we got out of the car I called his bluff and said: 'You can bring your bag now because I want to go up to the flat and change before dinner.' He looked at me in a complete state of panic and then pulled an overnight bag out of the boot – how funny. I was so happy because he was – still is – so sexy and I definitely wanted to bed him. We've been together for four years! ❞

Too much of a good thing?

If you do have sex on a first date, you must realise it will be difficult – nigh on impossible – to get back on the traditional path of courtship. Once you've put out, he may want to stay in. This may suit you too; after all sex is one of the most important parts of a relationship (anyone who denies this is lying or not having much sex). But the dinner and drinks out on the town may dry up while the 'nights in front of the television' (nudge, nudge, wink, wink) will flourish. Get cosy and make the most of new-relationship shagging but insist on at least going out for a few drinks before you hit the love den. You still need to get to know him.

Louise, 23

❝ How to rescue first dates? Sometimes sex is the answer. I had a first date a few months ago cunningly engineered by me pretending to be helpless and asking: 'Can you show me round Streatham?'

Here's how it went:

- ◆ 7.30 p.m. My dream date meets me at the station.

- ◆ 8.30 p.m. I'm tipsy.

- ◆ 9.30 p.m. I can't stand.

- ◆ 10.30 p.m. He reveals he supports Arsenal; I'm a Spurs fan.

- ◆ 10.31 p.m. I call him a wanker.

- ◆ 10.32 p.m. He is very offended.

- ◆ 10.33 p.m. I grab him and snog the face off him.

- ◆ 10.40 p.m. I am forgiven; we get a cab back to his.

- ◆ Three months on: we're still having mind-blowing, passionate sex.'

Midnight runs

The actual 'art of love-making' as your mother might call it will be discussed in later chapters, but for now we need to discuss the logistics of having sex when you didn't expect to. We can assume – being a modern girl on a date – you would have shaved, matched and moisturised so you won't be too worried about removing your clothes. But after first-date sex, one can feel incredibly uncomfortable. What do you do now? You've just shown a virtual stranger bits of your body your doctor hasn't seen and now you're struggling to make conversation. Do you sit, or sleep, through it? Pretending to doze off while he fidgets, snores, wheezes – or even worse stays awake – could be difficult. Stay if you fancy doing it again, and again, and again (as long as you haven't got an early meeting which you need to be alert for) or if the idea of getting dressed, going out and finding a way home is too distressing. If you know staying is futile, get out of there as quickly as is polite. You can't put a price on sleeping in your own bed, not having to worry about farting and/or dribbling in your sleep, and having your favourite moisturiser and shampoo for the morning. Enjoy the afterglow for all of 30 minutes before explaining you have a busy day tomorrow and you really should get home. He'll probably be grateful to have his bed to himself too.

> **NB Should he stay or should he go?** If you've lured him back to your place, it may be harder to get rid of him. It might be less stressful to let him stay, in which case you should offer him a towel – and definitely offer him coffee in the morning. It would be rude not to. If you can't bear the thought of him cuddling you all night, be upfront about it. Say you never let people stay over on first dates (he may think your morals are a bit warped but hey-ho!) and ask him if you should book him a taxi. Again, he may grateful for an easy escape route. Wanting to do a runner is not a bad sign – unless the thought of spooning him makes you nauseous – it means you've got to get to know each other and you've got busy lives. You're independent individuals and that's cool.

The end?

Whether your first date ends before midnight in a bar, or at the bus station the following morning, you need to make a lasting impression if you want to see him again. It's obvious you got on incredibly well (you laughed, learnt and leaned in for a kiss) but the bit where you say goodbye is always a bit embarrassing. On departure, he should say he'll call. If he doesn't it isn't that there won't be a second date – maybe he thinks it's obvious that there will be. If you feel confident, tell him to call you. If he paid for the date remember to say thank you – and perhaps follow up with an email the following afternoon.

NB The three-day rule. A modern man waits on average three days after a first date to make contact. If he calls the next day, you're well in there girl. He knows you're a busy, popular girl and he has to book you far in advance. Oh what it is to be wanted! If he leaves it longer than three days, he's being a bit too nonchalant and is either waiting for a better option, multi-dating, or no longer interested. If he calls you after three days with an explanation about a sick parent, business trip, or broken leg, forgive him and arrange a second date.

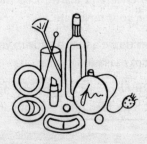

Secrets of Success

◆ If you have to cancel a first date, give the boy as much notice as possible. Not so he can rebook with someone else from his little black book but so he knows you are polite. If possible, try to rearrange the date while you have him on the phone. If the reason for your cancellation means your next few days are in turmoil, ask for his patience and promise him your next free night.

◆ Arrange to meet inside a venue if possible – it's warmer, there are toilets and drinks available. Take a magazine in case he's running late. Reading a book may look a bit serious.

◆ It isn't a proper first date if there's more than two of you. Don't accept an invite to meet his family. Tread carefully if your first date is as his guest at a family wedding. It happens more than you'd think.

◆ Never accept a first date that lasts longer than 24 hours. It may turn into a weekend-long love-in but you need an escape clause. Trips abroad are not good.

◆ Always look your date in the eye – anything else will be seen as disinterest.

◆ If he takes you to an unbearable venue, like to watch his favourite football team play, cope with good grace. Put it down to experience and learn to be more forthcoming with suggestions on your next date.

◆ Never take friends on a first date with you or call your mother mid-date. It looks very immature.

◆ It is rude to phone or text anyone during a first date. As soon as you've met him, turn off the phone if possible.

- If there are awkward silences, don't be tempted to waffle on about nothing. Ask him a question about himself – most men can talk about themselves for hours.

- Do not make eyes at cute guys across the room in his company.

- Try not to be put off by one flaw. Sometimes it's hard to overlook bad shoes, poor taste in music or an embarrassing surname (Bottom, Willey, Slowcock, Pratt et al) but if it's only one thing you find annoying, stay the distance to see if you can overlook it.

- If he's asked you out for dinner, eat. Nothing is more offputting than a girl pushing a salad leaf around the plate. And psychologists say the more a person enjoys food and drink, the more she enjoys sex... what a great excuse to go for the three courses.

- Drink but don't get to the room-spinning stage. Follow every three glasses of booze with a glass of water.

- Don't let him order for you (although let him choose the wine if he knows more about it than you) and try not to order the same thing. It could seem a little pathetic.

- Make sure your friends haven't made plans to go to the same place. He'll think there's a conspiracy.

- Don't eat with your mouth open.

- If he makes a nervous romantic gesture – like calling over the violinist or buying you a red rose – don't automatically think he's tacky. He just doesn't know you very well yet. If he starts serenading you, however, run like the wind.

- If it's cold outside and he offers his jacket, don't say no. He's being thoughtful.

- Be prepared. Take an umbrella if it looks like rain. Drowned rats are unattractive.

- If you're a smoker and he's not, wait until after the meal to light up – and ask first. Not for permission but for politeness' sake.

- Don't talk through the film, show, concert – save your comments for the interval. This may be his pet hate.

- If your date insists on paying for dinner and drinks, let him. He's not being sexist; he's being polite. However, some men are nervous about insulting modern girls or are quite mean, so do always take some cash with you. If you suspect that he's tight, don't date him again.

- If you asked him out on the date, you should offer to pay. He'll probably refuse but be pleased you offered.

- Under no circumstances should you tell a guy you love him on a first date. Neither should you mention you're being sued by your former employer, you love Meatloaf or you can burp 'Wannabe' by the Spice Girls.

- First-date sex is only acceptable if you know the odds that it will be a one-night stand and are prepared to take the risk. If you fancy him but can't see it being a long-term thing, consider it a dating experience with a bonus at the end.

- Be prepared. Always carry a condom. Even if you have contraceptive coverage for pregnancy, don't take the risk of catching something nasty. Don't assume the man will carry condoms.

- If you don't want to sleep with him, say no and don't feel guilty. Men can be very persuasive – especially when it's a 'nightcap' or a one-hour trip through the rain on a bus to your cold, clothes-covered flat. Mentally fast-forward to the morning... Will you regret it?

◆ Don't cry if he doesn't want to stay the night.

◆ Don't carry on drinking alcohol after 2 a.m. – you'll feel lousy.

◆ If you do fancy first-date sex, go for it. Don't think of what your parents, priest or prudish colleague would say. Why do people think it's acceptable for men to enjoy sex while women should wait for it?

◆ In a bid to look beautiful, who could blame you if your abode now looks more like a department store after an earthquake than a seduction palace. If you think there's a chance you might be coming back to yours to get it on later and your home is an embarrassment, be sure to spend a few minutes shoving stuff in cupboards and spraying air freshener. Remove dirty knickers, plates and magazines. Do not pick up a Hoover. A girl should ignore household appliances on first-date days.

◆ When he asks you for a second date, if you are genuinely busy for the next few weeks, set a firm date so he knows that he's not being rejected.

◆ If he looks great the morning after – and you have sex again after breakfast – he's a keeper.

◆ Love – and lust – at first date does exist. Enjoy it and don't let anyone tell you otherwise.

◆ Remember at all times, however apprehensive you're feeling, he'll be just as nervous. Sometimes it's better to acknowledge it so you can both let your guard down. It might be the icebreaker you need.

Chapter Nine

Let's get serious

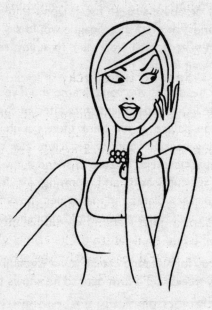

THERE WAS AN INSTANT attraction, the first date went well... and now you are confident he could be around for a while. You haven't quite booked the church yet but you're happy to think he could decorate your tree with you at Christmas.

Setting the pace

You may be in love with him after the first date but try to take things slowly. Do not sit in every night praying for him to call. Do not forget who your friends are because you are so interested in getting to know his. Do not forget to feed your cat because you haven't been home for five days. Limit dates to three per week in the first month. Any more than that and those around you will think you've turned into a one-track-minded limpet. And you're setting yourself up for a fall if it all goes pear-shaped.

Second time lucky

The first date is normally held on mutual, safe ground. It involves alcohol, sometimes food (although this can be tricky) and a limited time span, just in case you don't get on. After a successful first date, two or three similar dates can be arranged. Stick to a winning formula so you both feel comfortable, for example, a new bar without a history for either of you, or a quiet restaurant equidistant between your homes. You could even return to the venue where you first met. There are several reasons why the second, third and fourth dates are just as important as the first:

◆ You liked each other physically the first time – can you imagine being attracted to each other long-term?

◆ Without 'first-night' nerves, you can relax and let your guard down a little. Will he like the more relaxed, real you?

◆ You can get to know a little more about him, his history and his intentions (don't be too pushy on these matters though).

◆ You have more time to discuss other interests, and can start to see if you share similar taste in music, food, film etc.

◆ You can have a rerun of the first kiss and understand if it really was as kneewobbling as you thought it was.

It is never acceptable on a second date to:

◆ bring a friend;

◆ take him to a family event, or be expected to attend one as his partner;

◆ introduce him to people as your boyfriend if you bump into an acquaintance;

◆ get rollicking drunk and tell him you think you'll marry him;

◆ discuss how good you are in bed, how many people you've slept with, or your penchant for rubber;

◆ expect him to pay for everything if he paid on the first date;

◆ be late and not phone to apologise, assuming you don't have to make an effort anymore;

◆ not wash or brush your teeth. At this stage physical appearance is still the most important thing;

◆ be rude. He'll still be nervous so pay him a genuine compliment and remind him of what a great time you had on your first date;

◆ forget the first-date rules. You haven't won him over yet.

When you first start dating, it should only be about that. Dating. Enjoy the intrigue and flirting and don't expect too much. Everyone has past experiences that will make him or her wary or shy of meeting a new love. Don't be disappointed if he doesn't fit your ideal immediately. Work at it.

Not so lucky

What happens between a successful first, second, or third date and him not calling you again to make your man, er, not call you again? Many modern girls believe it's because men are born with a non-negotiable fear of commitment and they're probably right – it's got nothing to do with you or your penchant for cheesy pop music. Men are scared because they assume as soon as they get into a new relationship, their friends without relationships will be having more fun than them. Are they right?

Men can suffer from this all their lives. Even married men assume that all unmarried blokes lead lives of heady, er, hedonism with lapdancers, Brazilian supermodels and air hostesses. In fact, for most single men, the climax of a typical evening is watching a rerun of *Only Fools and Horses* while eating baked beans and drinking beer. (This is also true of married men, although statistically they are far more likely to heat the baked beans first.)

This is why, when a guy goes out on a date with a woman and finds he really likes her, he will often worship her from afar and avoid her for the rest of his life. The bloke has realised if he takes you out again, he'll probably like you even more. (Male logic!) Eventually he'll fall in love, get married, have children, then grandchildren. He'll fall into a life of slippers, cocoa and his waist will expand considerably. On his 60th birthday, the pair of you will be flying to a distant land to celebrate, sipping champagne and reminiscing about your younger days... when a gaggle of lapdancers, Brazilian supermodels and air hostesses ask him to initiate them into the Mile High Club. And he'll have to say no because he's married to you!

Is it love he's after or just a good time?

After five or six dates, it might be worth taking stock to see if you're on the same track. You might be besotted but if he's only looking for a stopgap until he emigrates to Africa, you could be left broken-hearted. Likewise, you may have bewitched him into the idea of marriage but if you're just looking for a social life with sex, you're being unfair. Your wider plans shouldn't really be discussed but listen out for the warning bells... there will be plenty of them.

He's looking for a serious girlfriend if:

◆ he asks you to help decorate his flat;

◆ he thinks it's important you get on with his sister;

◆ all of his family and friends seem to know everything about you;

◆ he calls your mum and dad, well, Mum and Dad;

◆ he offers to insure you on his car;

◆ he offers joint babysitting services to friends in a bid to make you broody;

◆ he buys you jewellery;

◆ he talks about booking a holiday;

◆ he talks about Christmas, next Valentine's Day etc;

◆ he buys you a wide-screen television or stereo (because he assumes he'll get use out of it too at some stage).

He's looking for a fun girl to have regular sex with if:

◆ he encourages you to go out with your mates;

◆ he encourages your mates to go out with his mates;

◆ he's always busy on Friday nights;

◆ he hasn't suggested a week away, only a dirty weekend;

◆ he only comes to your place for food or sex;

◆ he buys you flowers from a petrol station, not a florist;

◆ he feels sorry for people with children;

◆ no one will ever be as good a cook as his mum;

◆ he watches reruns of *Baywatch*;

◆ he has more fun with your body than your brain.

Both of these men have their place in time but know what you are dealing with. You'll either be dumped for being needy or branded a cruel, cold bitch for toying with his affections.

When do you stop 'seeing' and start 'being'?

Humans like to label things – it helps us to understand what's going on around us. When we first start dating someone, describing what's going on to others can be tricky. Are you just dating, enjoying someone's company, seeing each other, or going out together? One small flip-out with the vocabulary and you're transported back to snogging teens or your mother goes to buy a hat. So when are you officially boyfriend and girlfriend?

Firstly, if he asks you to be his girlfriend, try to think he's cute rather than immature. Okay, so up to now you thought only seven-year-old boys who are looking for playground kudos ask this but maybe he's nervous and likes you a lot. Forgive him. You should not ask to be his girlfriend though. He might think you're desperate and a bit *Sweet Valley High*.

The following are the clearest signs you have hit the girlfriend cusp:

♦ You've been on more than 5 dates.

♦ You've met his friends but not his family.

♦ He lets you pay for a few drinks on a date.

♦ He starts to tell you a few bad stories about himself.

♦ He doesn't know how to introduce you anymore when you're out (suddenly just your name won't do and he certainly won't refer to you as his friend).

♦ He accidentally uses a baby voice in your presence.

♦ He suggests you go out during the day.

♦ You call him at work and his colleagues seem to know who you are when you leave a message.

This is the fun stage of dating. You're both keen – if a little unsure – and trying to be on your best behaviour while revealing your true character. You may even have farted in front of him by this stage (by accident of course) and he thought it was quite sweet. When he buys you a toothbrush to keep at his place, you know you're in it for the medium-to-long-term.

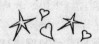

Introducing him to your past

After a few dates, you will wish to know about each other's exs. Not to pry and analyse but just to understand what you do and don't like. When doing your Hercule Poirot bit, ask general details about how long they dated, if they lived together, why it finished, but don't demand to know favourite sexual positions, why he fell in love with her or if he still misses her. You won't like the answers, whether they are good or bad. Likewise, you should answer basic questions about your past boyfriends but don't go into detail about your ex-fiancé's aftershave, post-coital routine or 'your song'. If you have been married before and/or have children, tell him on the second date. This is a real past.

Sharing your sexual history

Tread carefully when he starts to ask you about your past sexploits. You may be desperate to know how many women he has slept with and how good they were. You may even want to know if he's ever slept with a prostitute, if he's into anal sex or if he's ever had a gay experience. But do remember, if you pry and he answers, he'll expect the same from you. You should be honest if possible. A modern girl with decorum should fear nothing about her past. But we've all had a few dodgy moments so feel free to omit those (three-in-a-beds, sleeping with minors, ugly one-night stands) from a prospective boyfriend – they're fun to remember on nights out with the girls but he might think differently.

If you've slept with over ten people, also feel free to whip out your artistic licence. At least until he's told you how many people he's shagged. If it's over fifty, however, never admit it. Even I'm shocked – you have been busy. If he's slept with over fifty, you should of course be equally disturbed. He sounds like a one-man condom testing machine (let's hope!).

If you've only slept with one person, tell him. Men love feeling special and this will make him feel practically unique. Don't play the creepy schoolgirl-virgin card, just be upfront about your choosiness and when you do decide to sleep with him, it will be extra special. Don't assume he's a goon if he's only slept with one person. Men can be picky too. And practice doesn't make perfect. A man who has only had a few serious relationships will normally be better in bed than the local one-night stand champion.

Joanna, 35

❝ I met an RAF pilot on a fairly drunken St Patrick's Day in Mayfair. He wasn't really my type, but he pursued me, telling me about his BMW Z3 and how lonely he was up at his base during the week. After about three weeks of dating and getting to like him more and more, one thing finally led to another and we went to bed. Afterwards, he started quizzing me about my sexual history – how many, where, when, had I ever picked up someone and slept with them on the first date, etc. Well, as a fun-loving girl, I had nothing to hide, or so I thought! So I told him everything. Big mistake. He dropped me like a hot potato, saying that I didn't meet his standard of 'honour and integrity', and if I was such a goer, he was angry that I had made him wait three weeks! I was pretty devastated by this but got my revenge a year later when my phone rang and a girl said: 'You don't know me, but do you know Neal Willey?' I said I had dated him for a month last year but it didn't work out. She said: 'I have been his girlfriend for a year, and I just found a book with girls' names listed, and I'm calling them one by one to check up on him – and he slept with every single one of them!' Honour and integrity, indeed, Captain Willey. However, I did learn a very valuable lesson – NEVER tell your boyfriend about your past sexual exploits – there is nothing to be gained, and he will only think less of you, and will use it against you. Make him think he's the only one – men like to think women are innocent. **)**

If either of you are virgins, don't push anything. Take it slowly. Sex is bad unless both of you are confident, comfortable and turned-on. Too soon and it could put one of you off for – well, not life – but definitely a few years.

NB If he can't let it go let him go. If he constantly refers to past relationships or sexual choices, think seriously if you want to be with this man. Distrust, bitterness or mockeries are not good blocks on which to build a healthy relationship.

Reality check

It's not just your past relationships and sexual conquests that could put him off. Here are some other things about the real you that could scare him – so introduce them carefully, quietly and without a chip on your shoulder. Everyone has their problem areas, so be careful in case you hit his. There's no accounting for taste.

◆ Don't tell him about electrolysis, or waxing to remove moustaches, hairy chests or problem pubic hair until you're engaged.

- ◆ Don't share the trials of IBS.

- ◆ Play down your webbed feet, missing finger, glass eye or metal skull until you know he's sympathetic and intelligent about such matters.

- ◆ If you are a dyed ginger, tell him before he sees you without make-up on or start dyeing your lashes and brows. If you're ginger and proud, stay cool.

- ◆ If you used to be 30 stone, wait a little longer to show him your fat-phase picture. He should admire your will power but he may be scared to leave you alone with his fridge.

A bird in the hand...

It is about the time that you share histories, you realise this could be a guy worth pursuing – at the rejection of all others. At some point a girl has to make a decision. When you're free and single it's fine to have university friends who you snog occasionally, colleagues who you flirt with on work nights out, and the hanger-on ex who is there for comfortable sex when your dry spell is sending you round the bend. And sadly, it's too often the case that men are like buses – you wait for a decent one for months and then three come together. But sigh no more ladies, sigh no more. There are lots of Mr Right Nows about and you have to commit to Mr Right.

If you have reached a decision stalemate regarding two or more men, ask yourself these questions:

- ◆ Who has tried to change me the least?

- ◆ Who seems proud when they introduce me to friends and family?

- Whose email makes me smile the most first thing in the morning?

- When I see which one of their phone numbers on my mobile, do I shiver with excitement?

- Who has bought me something so perfect (however small) I could have chosen it myself?

Do not choose one man over the other on account of:

- salary;

- status;

- class;

- size of penis;

- ability to speak foreign languages.

However, the following factors are all seemingly traditional and shallow but need to be evaluated if this relationship is to be a long and prosperous one:

- Do I like his family?

- Do I trust him with money?

- Do I trust him with my attractive friends?

- Do we share similar views on politics, ethics, religion etc?

- Do we seem compatible in bed?

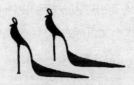

Obviously, once you pick one man to date above another, you will always wonder what could have been. So just after you've decided which one to go for, make a list of all the failed Romeo's problems, annoying habits and dodgy moments. While you are still seeing the victor, refer to this list in brief moments of doubt.

Exclusivity

If you're willing to commit and stop dating others, he should do the same. There's no point in you forsaking all others if he's still the wildest man on the streets of your town. Some couples – even married ones – insist that open relationships work. Maybe, but only if you don't suffer from jealousy, stress, hurt, regret and intimacy issues. The great thing about being in a relationship is the way the other person makes you feel: adored, worshipped, loved, and honoured. If they're off doing it with every Tanya, Donna or Harriet, you're not going to get the nice sensations – just the snoring, dirty socks and arguments over who holds the remote control. Decide early on if you both want to be exclusive.

NB Don't burn all your bridges. You seem pretty certain at the moment who you should date but fast-forward a few months, or even years. If things don't work out and you're still single, it would be good to phone or bump into some guys who nearly made the grade before. They could have improved and you'll kick yourself if they won't give you the time of day because you dumped them cruelly before.

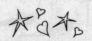

Warning bells

Don't ignore the warning bells. If he's not returning your calls, not looking you in the eye, staying out late, going on lots of business trips, not introducing you to his friends – be careful. I'm not saying he's scum but the first few months of a relationship are the most passionate, and if he can't be arsed to make an effort now, be careful.

Keeping your feet on the ground

Unfortunately, not everyone will be as happy as you and your mother that your love life is going so well. You should learn to show off and flounce about only when amongst close comrades who you won't offend. Be sensitive to those who have just lost a partner, or the singles that are still worried about the shelf and sitting on it.

How not to annoy your friends

When you get a new boyfriend – especially if a relationship is quite a novel experience for you – you will soon descend into mush mode. You'll dream about him, smile when you think of him, laugh at little adventures you've had together when you're with other people, and doodle his name all over your newspaper. Try not to be too Sandra Dee-ish. No one likes a wet blanket, least of all a group of fantastic modern girls who can see their fellow fabulouso being sucked into soppy school. Prove to your mates you are still cool by:

◆ not blowing them out last-minute for your new man;

◆ not texting him when you go out to coffee for a gossip;

- allowing conversation to flow without: 'New bloke says...';

- sparing them the details of his anatomy;

- sparing them the details of how many times you had sex last night;

- not offering to fix them up with his mates unless they ask;

- not bringing him along to girls-only nights;

- not wearing his rugby shirt and sniffing it intermittently while Saturday shopping;

- paying an interest in their lives, men or no men.

How not to annoy your boss

The less committed you are to a man, the more committed you're likely to be to your company. It's true in the first flushes of love, you can't get out the door quick enough... and then you crawl in half an hour late in the morning and proceed to stare out of the window all day long. You can prove to your boss you're still professional in the following ways:

- Getting to work on time; it might be tough to drag yourself away from lover boy but there'll be plenty more mornings. Set the alarm half an hour earlier than usual to fit in a quick tussle if that's what's making you late.

- Limiting hangovers to the weekend. Beer breath in meetings is so uncool (once a month is understandable, just keep painkillers, water and sausage sandwiches next to you at all times).

- Not sharing details of your sex life with your colleagues because they are just that. Colleagues, not friends or relationship experts.

- Not taking more sick days to lounge about in bed. Your boss will put two and two together and make sex-crazy chick.

- Not sidetracking studying for a professional qualification because you'd rather be with your new guy. Keep motivated, even if it means studying in your lunch hour.

- Not taking the piss on the phone or with email. One call a day maximum.

- Not allowing your new guy to hang around reception for you all day long. You won't be able to concentrate.

Dating drawbacks

It's not all hearts and flowers in the land of new relationships. Only you'll know if he's worth it. At times, love can be:

- Stressful. (Does he like me? When can I see him? Is he serious about me?)

- Time-consuming. (When can I wash my hair, shave my legs, or visit my grandma? I don't want to commute between my flat and his flat!)

- Freedom-reducing. (Do I have to see him on Saturdays? What if I fancy the new guy at work? What if I want to go on holiday with my mates?)

- Humiliating. (I'm speaking like a baby and singing into a hairbrush – am I mad or just in the first throes of love?)

◆ Stupefying. (What do you mean there's an economic crisis going on? All I want to know is if my bum looks big in this – I've got a date tonight!)

But on the plus side...

You get to flirt, dance, dream, talk, gossip, laugh, joke, smile, kiss, cuddle, share, hope, thrill, play and love. You also – unless you're terribly old-fashioned and planning on saving yourself for your wedding night – get to have lots of sex.

Getting back in the saddle

You may not have been very busy in the bedroom department for quite some time, so blow away the cobwebs with some pelvic tricks and sexy tips guaranteed to give you confidence (and hopefully an orgasm) every time you take your clothes off... and while we're on the subject – he's not thinking how large your thighs are or how small your boobs are the first time he sees you naked. He's thinking: 'Wow – I'm bloody lucky.' Confidence and enjoyment are the sexiest things in the world, so try not to feel worried. Enjoy yourself. Don't think: 'No way, José, I can't go on top, my stomach will hang out.' Think: 'Why not – he really fancies me and I'm more likely to have an orgasm on top, that's what it says in *Cosmopolitan*.' You go, girl.

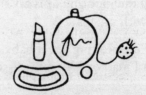

> **NB It's better to be safe than sorry.** Sex is fun and can make you feel fantastic, but it can also make you feel terrible. Use condoms. It's not embarrassing to whip one out and demand he puts it on – you're saving yourselves a lot of trouble (until you know where he's been, play safe).

Fail-proof seduction section

Get him in the mood for a long night ahead. Here's how:

◆ When you're at dinner, accidentally flash him a bra strap or cross your legs slowly to show you're not wearing any knickers. Vixen-laydee...

◆ Arms-over-the-head stretch. This catlike manoeuvre awakens him to your breasts (which you're virtually shoving in his face) flexibility and your long arms.

◆ Whisper breathily into his ear (the old ones are the best).

◆ Laugh seductively, not like a drain with flu.

◆ Touch yourself; don't scratch yourself. Gently rest fingers on your collarbone.

◆ Ask him to take a shower or bath with you.

◆ Offer him a massage.

◆ Cook him his favourite dinner (but don't overfeed him or he'll fall asleep) and pour him his favourite drink.

◆ Turn off the television, sit down wrapped up together and talk.

◆ Buy a rug and suggest an indoor picnic.

> **NB Limit date preparation to yourself.** Don't spend hours plumping cushions on your bed, plucking any stray hair on your being, spraying your home, car, or body with pheromone sprays, get blisters strutting about in shag-me boots or lighting candles throughout your flat. If it's that hot, he won't notice the external effort you've made – only you (and that's the way you want it!).

Sex for men

Obviously everyone wants different things in the sack. The world would be a very boring place if we all wanted missionary-position intercourse, once a week for ten minutes. Although saying that, the majority of women do want missionary-position intercourse, once or twice a week for ten minutes. I'm sure the dominatrixes among you will think this is terribly dull, but most women find it emotionally fulfilling.

Sexual healing?

No sex life is without its difficulties – especially when you've just started dating and getting to know each other. Here are a few common dilemmas and how to handle them:

◆ If your man is more king prawn than porn king... if he's a bit petite in the downstairs area, make the most of fore-play. Don't make him any more insecure about it than he already is (this will affect performance). He'll be aware of his downfall and this will probably make him more agile and energetic with his tongue and hands.

◆ If your man is more King Kong than ding-dong... go on top. You can control the speed and depth and jump off easily if he gets too carried away. Use a lubricant if necessary and beware of thrush and cystitis. Harsh sex can cause these nasty problems.

◆ If your man is enjoying himself a bit too much... and comes too quickly, get him to change positions frequently (this slows things down a bit) and try pressing your finger on his perineum.

◆ If your man is a little too vocal... tell him to whisper in your ear, and that you can't concentrate on getting the best orgasm ever while he's wailing and laughing like a hyena. If he makes animal noises or speaks like a cartoon character, get your clothes on and leave immediately.

◆ If your man can't get an erection... lay off and ask him to pleasure you some other way, or to watch while you do it yourself. If he's still agitated, sleep on it and try again in the morning. If the problem persists – and you've talked through any emotional issues that might be hanging around in his head – go to a doctor. There are really good tablets to combat this problem.

◆ If your man can't make you come... give him a few tips – subtly. Don't bark instructions, you'll scar him for life. Lead his hand to places you want to be touched, say: 'Don't stop' if you want him to carry on, and introduce sex toys for both of you to enjoy if you need to. Never exclude him.

If your man doesn't like sex, try to change his mind. Seduce him. Savour him. If it's still not working, understand you can have a close, committed relationship without frequent sex. If, however, he's leaving you so unsatisfied you're starting to look elsewhere, get out. Sex is important and it is an indication of how good your future looks. Sex counsellors admit if you're making love less than once a week, you're on the danger list.

If your man is making dangerous sexual demands, tell him to stop. Go as far as you feel comfortable, even if others may think it a little strange, and he shouldn't push you any further. If he does something to scare, hurt or damage you, tell him where to go. Let him go play on his own.

Jill, 35

❝ When I first started dating my husband, we had a really rough time in bed. Well, not rough in a passionate, aggressive way – but rough in a difficult way. He couldn't keep an erection for longer than a few minutes. As soon as we turned attention away from him and on to me, he seemed to lose it. At first, this really upset me. I assumed it was because he was selfish and used to only satisfying himself. We argued a few times until eventually he admitted it was because he liked me so much I made him nervous. I was so relieved. We both loosened up, even laughed about it, and after a few efforts, we went the distance. Girls should remember there's lots of pressure on the boys too – it's not just about the girls being thin enough. ❞

Secrets of Success

◆ Don't count your chickens before they've hatched, i.e. don't tell everyone that you've met your future husband... when you've only been on three dates. He may be the one for you, but be discreet in the early stages.

◆ If you suspect he's just having fun, but you're falling for him fast, it may be wise to distance yourself. There's nothing worse than falling in love with someone who warned you they were just up for a fling.

◆ If his friends tell you he talks about you all the time, it's serious. Men don't lose street cred with their mates over just anyone.

◆ Try to play down your David Beckham obsession until the fifth date – by then he'll feel comfortable enough to tell you he loves him too.

◆ When you've stayed over at his place three or more times – and you're still getting on well – it's acceptable to keep a toothbrush and a clean pair of knickers there. Don't move in lock, stock and barrel though. Bringing your favourite mug and your winter wardrobe on your fourth visit will freak him out.

◆ Buy him presents if you want to... keep them thoughtful, playful and reasonably priced. No diamonds yet. And you shouldn't expect them before the six-month mark either (unless he's a millionaire playboy and he buys them for everyone – even his cleaner).

◆ Save your sparkling sarcasm until the third or fourth date – and warn him about it. Men don't like bitches, generally.

- Don't try and fix up your mate with his mate until you're a bit steadier. It would be hard to handle if you lost your love, and your friend still went out with him socially thanks to you.

- Going away for the weekend is a great step forward after a handful of dates. You'll get time to see him in holiday mode (if only for one or two days) – and get ready to go out together, which is a great relationship leveller.

- If he's moving too fast, go away with your girlfriends for a few days.

- Don't offer your friends his cancelled slots in your diary. They'll soon pick up on what you're doing and get upset about it. You'll need their support when you have your first argument with dream-lover.

- Minimise the information you pass on to your parents. They'll get over excited and store every piece of information for the next 50 years. There's nothing like paternal approval to put a dampener on a sexy fling.

- Beware if he asks to borrow money, move in with you or meet your very attractive friend on his own when you've only been dating a few months.

- Also beware of the man who says he loves you before you've been on five dates. He probably says it to all the ladies and can't think of a more original seduction line.

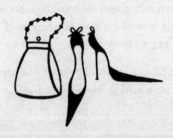

- Don't believe a man who shows off about his sexual prowess before you've tried him out. If he were really good, he wouldn't need to sell himself.

- It's perfectly acceptable for a modern girl to keep condoms in her handbag at all times. Be prepared.

- Even if you do go back to his flat for coffee, you don't have to have sex. A girl can say no whenever she wants. No means no, and she shouldn't be made to feel guilty for it.

Chapter Ten

From dating to eternity?

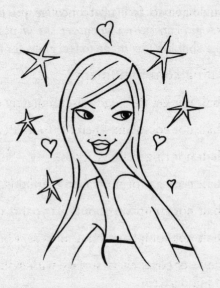

I S LIFE EVER EASY? Well, love life – no. You see getting the man is quite difficult. Keeping him is a little harder. And then still wanting him after three months of drunken gropes, disgusting eating habits and an inability to see the merits of *Sex and The City* is practically impossible. Maybe you were better off on your own?

The panic period

Relax, laydeez. When you first start dating someone, this period of panic is completely normal and easily explainable.

You're dedicating a lot of time to someone you've only just met. Perhaps you're dreaming about moving in, marrying and maybe even procreating with the guy. No wonder you're nervous. I'm surprised you're able to read – you should be shaking, breaking out in nervous sweats and screaming 'no, no, no'. When you first get into a new relationship, you have to face up to new responsibilities and restrictions.

The ten dating commandments

1. Thou shalt not get to snog indiscriminately anymore.

2. Thou shalt not complain when the football is on.

3. Thou shalt not ring ex-boyfriends.

4. Thou shalt not nag for no reason (period is no excuse).

5. Thou shalt not complain about dirty pants on floor.

6. Thou shalt not complain about toilet seat being left up.

7. Thou shalt not cover every surface with make-up, magazines and underwear.

8. Thou shalt not be allowed to go to bed with a book before 11 p.m.

9. Thou shalt not hold the remote control while he is in the house.

10. Thou shalt not criticise his mother, even if she's hellish.

All of these rules are surmountable, though. You will have to change your lifestyle if you choose to have a relationship but there are lots of bonuses too. Who needs a wee-free toilet seat when there's sex-on-tap to be had? Honestly, give it a few weeks of a free taxi service when you're out too late with your mates and you won't even notice the pizza boxes stacking up underneath the sofa. It's all give and take, and sometimes you will feel like you're giving more... but at other times (when you're premenstrual, watching a weepy movie or just got off the phone from your mother), he'll certainly be giving more. When you do feel annoyed, try to laugh it off. In relationships, laughter always is the best medicine.

When a few weeks of dates goes nowhere?

Sometimes – as promising as the first few dates are – one of you decides to stop calling. It's difficult to admit you can't make someone feel something they don't feel... but you can't. If it's him who cools things down, take comfort that it's probably nothing you did or didn't do. More likely he has pre-set ideas of what he wants from a woman and how committed he can be at that time.

If you are convinced you're got something worth saving, take a back seat for a while – and then call or email him after a week or so. Don't demand explanations, grand gestures or sex. Keep it cool. If he sounds offish or doesn't return your message, try once more a few days later and then call it quits. If you still can't forget about him after a few months, get dressed up, grab your mates and visit his regular hangout. Ignore him for the first few hours, bewitch every other man in the room with your stunning good looks and flawless personality and then slowly make your way over to him. If he's dismissive or unfriendly, turn on your heel and sashay back to your more appreciative audience. Some men are blind to fabulousness. He's not worth the effort.

You looking at me?

Okay, before we get into the problems your new beau suffers from – and believe me they'll be plenty – let's have a look at your issues.

Are you selfish?

Do you object when he starts to feel a little too at home in your home? Does he get under your feet if he hangs around at the weekend, or asks to get insured on your car so you can share the driving on your weekend away? Do you want to slap the back of his head every time he helps himself to the content of your fridge? Easily solved. Set the boundaries early on, i.e. after a few dates, and tell him gently but firmly when he's overstepped the mark. You can't suddenly explode after months of secret seething and expect him to understand. He sees his familiarity as a term of endearment – to show you how comfortable he feels in your presence. Of course, he could also be being lazy because he can't be arsed to stock up his own fridge. If you think he's taking advantage – try playing him at his own game. Suggest you hang out at his house or use his car. If he doesn't like the idea, you have a problem. Neither of you are willing to share – like spoilt only children – so you obviously don't like each other enough.

Are you scared of commitment?

You wanted a relationship and now you've got one you feel like you're being strangled or slowly drowning? Do you cancel dates to go out and get steaming drunk with your best mates? Do you panic if he wants to stay over and take you to lunch after a night of passion? Do you get carried away and assume he wants to marry you when he hasn't even asked to meet your father yet? Whoa, lady. You're being a bit paranoid. What are you so scared of? Losing your mind, personality, freedom, ambition and friends. Okay, it's sometimes hard for independent modern girls to join a partnership but one should remember one thing. A good relationship liberates you to do whatever you want. A perfect partner could never trap you, just give you a stable springboard to bounce off in whatever direction you choose. In fact, now you don't have to waste time thinking about love and sex and can spend the extra hours on yourself.

Are you possessive?

Do you get jealous when he talks to the old lady in the newsagent's, or when he smiles at the barmaid in his local pub? Do you get stressed out if he goes out with his mates from work on a Thursday night and – God forbid – takes some clients to a lap-dancing club? Okay, so the lap-dancing club isn't the classiest of ventures for your new love to be getting into but men are men. You can't expect them to stop looking at women because they've fallen for you. You should expect them to stop asking for phone numbers, snogging or lusting after other girls... but you can be on a diet and still look at the menu. If you flip out every time he smiles at a lady, you're asking for trouble. He may contain it all for a few months, or years, but then one day he'll explode – a massive rage of hormones – and resent you brainwashing him into submission. You can still see the merits of Brad Pitt, can't you? You still flirt with the guy in accounts who smells nice? You know it doesn't mean anything to you but harmless fun. It's the same for him until he's proved you different. If you find lipstick on his collar, you have a reason to be possessive and you can dump him or put him on a leash. Not until then.

Are you an outrageously grumpy cow?

Do you snarl at his jokes? Moan when he strokes your freshly washed hair? Scream, 'Can you get out of my face you irritating fuckwit,' when he tries to get affectionate? If the answer to the any of the above is yes, sort yourself out, get yourself on some kind of anger management therapy, take up t'ai chi, or start necking some herbal supplements, because you're lucky he's hung about this long!

He's so not Mr Perfect

Okay, so you're grumpy, possessive, selfish and commitment-shy but he's not all sunshine and roses. In fact, you can put your crazy antics down to hormones or insecurity but he's just plain maddening. Some things are nature, some are nurture, and some things are just his bloody-mindedness; the most important thing to remember is that all men are difficult. A few are out and out bastards who should be locked up and kept away from decent women, but others are just having a hard time with life like the rest of us. Remember stress, personality clashes and just a bad day at the office can make the calmest of people annoying. Some things you can change or adapt to and others are a bit trickier to deal with.

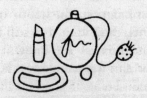

> **LISA,** 28
>
> ❝ My boyfriend from hell was a guy I'd met in Manchester one week and we'd had a fun few days together. He lived in Preston and I agreed to go up for the weekend to see how we'd get on long-term. I fell asleep on the train and ended up in Lancaster. I got to Preston two and a half hours late. He had the hump and we went to sleep in separate rooms without talking. The following morning, Princess Diana died. We talked for a little, got maudlin about life and had sex to depressing music on the BBC World Service. Within 24 hours I was as moody as him. ❞

Emotional issues

Where women almost enjoy crying, moaning, spilling and sulking, men shy away from sharing. It's some in-built caveman thang. They see opening up as a sign of weakness whereas women think they're hiding something. Not true – they just don't feel the need to discuss every second of inner turmoil with the world. Psychologists have finally proved that only two parts of the male brain (compared to nine parts of the female brain) are activated by emotional issues. This explains why men easily forget anniversaries, arguments and big emotional events. Men also have fewer electrical connections between the left and right side of the brain, so the flow of information is restricted. The right side is used to process emotion, the left to speak – which confirms men genuinely find it hard to articulate what they're feeling. So don't shout if he forgets your three-month anniversary or doesn't want to discuss last night's disagreement. He's a man.

Dirty dogs

Another peculiarity of man is his inability to wash or see dirt. Personal hygiene is often kept to a minimum and as for his flat... is it tidy? Do pigs fly? Not at his place, they're too busy wallowing about in their own shit. This is an easy dilemma to solve: tell him no clean teeth, armpits, and nether regions, no nookie. Refuse to go to his flat until he gets it sorted. If he hates cleaning or genuinely doesn't have the time, leave him the phone numbers of some good cleaners. Do not, I repeat, do not pick up a mop and start wiping. He'll expect you to do it all the time and soon prefer you to dust the lounge than go to bed.

> **NB Sharing duties.** Of course if you go on to get married and become a housewife, you should clean. There is nothing wrong with cleaning, only when it is taken for granted. If he works all day to support your family, he can expect a clean bath to soak in at the end of the day. Likewise, if you go out to work while he stays at home, he should become a Mr Mop.

The first time you meet his family...

The hardest thing about starting a new relationship is having to start a new relationship with lots of his relatives. Every family is different but here are some sure-fire rules:

◆ Don't push to meet the family too soon. All in good time. It's almost reassuring he doesn't bring all and sundry back to the ranch. When you do get invited, it's because you're you... special, like!

◆ Meeting for the first time is a minefield. Don't tell rude jokes at dinner. Don't joke about their little boy. Don't get drunk. Don't talk about your sexual preferences, what he's like in bed or about ex-boyfriends. Don't flirt with his dad. Don't wear revealing outfits, or dress too old for your years. Try not to spill anything or break the best plates. Offer to help in the kitchen. Bring a gift but don't make it too showy, or expensive – a bottle of wine, chocolates or flowers will do.

◆ Never slag off their children. They may know he is a scruffy monster but they don't need to hear it from you.

◆ Don't sulk if you're not the centre of attention.

◆ Don't argue if you have a different opinion – avoid the topics of politics, sex changes, West End musicals, racism and religion.

◆ Don't cancel attending a family do at the last minute. His mum could have gone to a lot of trouble on your behalf.

◆ Keep your party tricks for a party – don't offer to show his grandma your body-popping, gargling or moon-walking skills until you know them all quite well and know they won't hold it against you.

◆ Don't slag off his family. In a weak moment (after a fight) he may tell them what you said and your words will haunt your whole relationship.

◆ When they ask you about marriage, or the patter of tiny footsteps, grin and bear it. Don't assume your partner has hinted at these things to them.

◆ If you don't like them, be polite and courteous but don't make them a huge part of your life. Remain objective and they could grow on you.

◆ Don't try and get your families together until it's completely necessary i.e. an engagement party (yours!). You're asking for trouble.

> **KATE,** 29
>
> ❨ My boyfriend got completely hammered the night before meeting my mum for the first time… he was so nervous he thought he should drink his way into oblivion. On the morning of the meeting, he turned up looking as white as a ghost saying he had a stomach bug! My mum, being quite astute, had already guessed that he had a hangover, but I, being naïve, believed him! Mum had made a lasagne but halfway through the meal he ran to the kitchen sink and threw up. He apologised, I made excuses and my mum laughed – and in fact mentioned it in our wedding speeches. It made meeting his parents a lot easier, though. So my advice is, don't let nerves get the better of you the night before meeting the in-laws or pray he does something silly first. ❩

The first time you meet his friends…

The other bad thing about spending time with your new man is that you are expected to spend time with his friends. Friends are often as important as family – especially socially – so you need to make a good impression:

◆ Don't flirt with his friends inappropriately (if they have partners present, if you're all sober, if it upsets your boyfriend).

◆ Don't infiltrate their boys' nights (even if a few geezer-birds are in attendance). You wouldn't enjoy them anyway.

◆ Don't gatecrash weekends away with the boys – they want to play golf, fish, drink like fish, and not go on long country walks.

◆ Introduce his single mates to your single mates only if you think they'd get on and only if you can handle the stress of instigating new relationships.

◆ Don't moan about his friends unless you have a real issue, i.e. one put a hand on your arse, or stole money from your partner's wallet.

◆ Invite them over for dinner but don't expect their etiquette to be remarkable. They should bring a bottle and thank you for cooking, but they may revert to laddish behaviour over the lemon meringue.

◆ Everyone's different. Try not to take your difference of opinions too seriously.

◆ Remember – friends are a reflection of who someone is but not a mirror image. Don't sweat if you hate them all (just keep it to yourself).

The other women in his life

More than his moody side, you may find it difficult to accept he has other important ladies around him. Apart from his doting mother, you may expect to be number one on his lassie list without exception... only to discover he has a gaggle of fawning birds in the woodwork – just waiting to be cooed and fussed over. This isn't on, is it? Or is his ability to charm women of all ages (without the promise of sex) a sign that he is an all-round good guy?

Some women are acceptable – some should even be encouraged – and this is how you should handle them without jealousy or resentment. Remember, rather than making his female friendships a source of arguments, rejoice that they have probably taught him to be more in touch with his feminine side – and to get good gift advice.

The flatmate

If she's attractive, flirty, or one-of-the-lads, this is a horrible situation to be in. There are countless opportunities for them to get drunk and snog, or bump into each other while scantily clad across the breakfast table. On a date, she could call doing the damsel in distress thing and he might have to rush back to sort out the plumbing. And you may want to move in with him but he's tied into a contract with her.

How to handle her

Don't retaliate by moving yourself in wholesale – that's asking for trouble. Ask if she minds you staying over so often, check she doesn't mind you sharing her shampoo and buy her flowers if she's been cooking for you both. Don't make her feel like a stranger in her own home. Keep the gooseberry factor to a minimum (no snogging during

Frasier). View their living arrangement as the financial arrangement it obviously is... and be happy when you do get him to move in with you, he'll be house-trained.

The lingering ex

She sounds so glamorous – the ex. You've seen a few photos of her around his flat and you're nervous her arse is more toned than yours. His friends still ask how she is and he even refers to past holidays with a hint of nostalgia.

How to handle her
If the split was amicable, she's moved on but they still meet for a drink occasionally, you should handle this. They're grown-ups and he's committed to you. If she's still calling him all hours of the day and weeping down the phone, tell him this bothers you. But remember, don't be intimidated because he's with you – not her – and quite frankly she's acting like a loon. The more she stalks him, the more he'll run to you. Don't discuss her – she's not important enough to waste time on.

The overbearing sister

Around her, you can't get a word in edgeways. If she's not showing you pictures of lover boy exposing himself as a three-year-old, she's regaling you with tales of their strong bond and relationship with their parents. You find anything to do with your new man madly interesting, but you couldn't care less about his sibling.

How to handle her
Show an interest in their joint history – like his mum, you want to get her on your side. She cares a lot about her

brother so listen to her... but don't spend too much time around each other. While she's in the room, his attention will be split and he may take her advice a bit too seriously. Remember her birthday and you're sorted.

The chummy colleagues

These are the good-time girls who are always up for a swift pint after work and listen to his troubles over morning coffee. They flirt by the water cooler and may have even had a drunken snog at the Christmas party.

How to handle them
There's normally more than one – they tend to travel in packs – but the quickest way to win them over is to attend a few spontaneous piss-ups, slag off your boyfriend (jokingly of course) and pay an interest in them. Don't try to stop him going out with them (they'll get a lot of mileage out of this and take the piss out of your man) and appreciate the fact that if he fancied them, he could easily be dating one of them by now.

The man's woman

She understands the offside rule (we could too if we could be bothered), she goes to rugby matches and she can down a pint of lager in one. This is geezer-bird on steroids. One of the lads – she even goes to Ibiza with him and his male mates every summer. They share in-jokes, season tickets – and probably shaving foam (meow!).

How to handle her
Rest easy in the fact he doesn't find her sexy. He thinks she's a good laugh and he enjoys her company, but it stops there.

She might not be your kind of friend – modern girls don't need to act like a man or dismiss other women to be strong – so just wash your hair the nights he goes out with her.

Holiday from hell

Once you've been dating for a few months, you may want to go on holiday together. This can be a breeding ground for arguments – after all, it might be the first time you've spent prolonged periods of time together. Even if you live together, you have the office and friends to disappear to. On holiday, you'll have nothing, except the dodgy couple from Halifax you met on the camel ride, and the table tennis room. Not good options. Here's how not to kill each other:

◆ Pack your own suitcase. Don't rely on each other to know what you need.

◆ Plan where you are staying carefully. If he hates cities, don't insist on a trip to Los Angeles.

◆ Be sensible. Don't pack all your jumpers, 25 CDs and a Lilo – he may regret being a gentleman and offering to carry your case for you.

◆ If you didn't want to get to know each other better, you wouldn't be going away. So enjoy sharing a room, talking about preparing food, getting ready to go out together, washing up etc.

◆ Don't have any expectations. Go with the flow – especially if you're going to a hot country (tempers can flare when you're all sweaty).

◆ Don't hand him an itinerary at the airport. It's his holiday too.

- Don't cling to each other. Take a break, even if it's just soaking in the tub for two hours with a book.

- If one of you gets ill (which happens all the time on holiday) be sympathetic.

- Relax and enjoy each other's company.

- Maybe start with a weekend away, or at the most a week. A fortnight or a six-month tour of Australia is asking for trouble.

- We all act differently on holiday. He doesn't normally start drinking beer at midday so don't tell him off. You wouldn't be seen dead sipping a piña colada in a sombrero at home would you? No. So you are both letting your hair down. This means you're comfortable with each other, which is fab news.

JANE, 23

❝ Strange as it sounds, a bout of mutual food poisoning brought my man and me together on holiday. After dodgy paella, we got so sick we couldn't leave the apartment for three days. We got each other water, ran baths, battled our way to the chemist in the heat... and didn't even complain about the smell in the bathroom when the diarrhoea set in. We were too ill to have sex, so we talked and slept and read. We learnt a lot about how we both handle difficult situations – and liked each other more for it. ❞

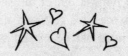

Twice the trouble

The biggest relationship-wrecker of all is finding out he's still seeing someone else. You've been faithfully and enthusiastically setting your sights on him while he's been setting his sights on a number of you. Should you cut your losses straight away or demand he makes a choice? Follow your heart because your head will instinctively tell you to back off. Your head is probably right – there'll be trust and insecurity issues to deal with – but if you've spent a few months with him and really like him, you could be cutting off your nose to spite your face. If you think it's worth the effort, ask him to choose and if he picks you, view that as the official start of your relationship.

If he refuses to commit or chooses the other girl, admit to yourself that he's not the right one for you. You can't commit to someone who doesn't put you first – he must be mad if he doesn't realise you're too good to lose after dating you for a few months.

LARA, 30

❝ I'd been sleeping with a guy at university for a few months – it was quite chummy and flirty and we never spoke about the future. One day, we were messing around, involving water fights and removal of clothing in his room in halls, when a girl, who I later found out to be his girlfriend, starts knocking on the door screaming for him to come out – she'd heard on the grapevine he was in there with someone. He told me to hide behind the en-suite shower curtain whilst he lowered himself out of the second-floor window and went round to meet his girlfriend at the front door and (eventually) convinced her he'd been out all evening and asked if she'd been waiting long. I could hear all this from the other side of the door and felt a bit stupid. The next time I saw him, I asked him to make a choice. He chose her so I moved on. No problem. I didn't want to be in the girlfriend's shoes in the future. 〟

Handling arguments

1. If you need to bring an issue up, think carefully beforehand what you want to achieve.

2. Minimise exaggeration, hysterics and dramatics.

3. If he upsets you, count to ten and try again.

4. Don't bring other people into arguments – even if friends and family want to get involved.

5. Stick to the argument – don't bring up past issues, which aren't relevant anymore.

6. Don't hit him (domestic violence towards men is increasing) and don't allow him to hit you. Not even once.

7. Try to keep the volume down. Not only will you scare the neighbours but also you won't be able to hear each other's point of views.

8. Once an argument is solved, forget about it. Don't hang on to the past.

9. If he won't confront your problems, write him a letter telling him how you feel and leave it with him to read when he's ready.

10. Remember that making up is so much fun. Arguing not only clears the air but can also bring a bit of passion back.

Enough is enough

Many problems are not solvable and you have to weigh up if it's worth it before you step up a gear and make your relationship more permanent. If you've tried to look on the bright side but aren't getting anywhere, it might be time to cut your losses. Work it out for yourself:

◆ Do you have more down moments than up moments?

◆ Are you are more stressed with him than happy?

◆ Are you settling because all your contemporaries have?

◆ Do you want to conform to society's expectations about girls of a certain age?

◆ Are you broody?

◆ Are your parents pressurising you to settle down?

◆ Do you want to have sex on tap and don't want to be labelled a slut by having frequent flings?

◆ Are you crap at DIY and/or car maintenance and feel you need 'a man around the house'? (Do a course.)

◆ Are you scared to dump the guy you've been seeing and he's keener than you are?

◆ Are you thinking financially, i.e. he's richer than you and drowns you in diamonds?

These aren't good enough reasons to spend time with someone. Turn back to chapter 1 and start again.

> **NB The comfort zone.** Once you have been living with someone for over two years, expect his or her annoying habits to grate a little more. It's not so much that the initial passion disappears, but it subsides into a lull of security, companionship and contentment. These are all good things too so don't panic. If you do have a brief 'what have I done?' period after being together for a while, ask yourself the questions above again. If your once-passionate relationship hasn't degenerated to a level of 'making do', you're still fine. No worries.

Spotting the signs of true intimacy

So how do you know when your relationship has turned from a sexy, fun fling into something more deep and meaningful? Basically, when it stops being just about sex and having fun. These things are still important but the more human side of both of you starts to come through as you let your guard down.

1. You may fart in your sleep and not care too much (although still get a bit red-cheeked when he reminds you with a whisper in your ear the next morning).

2. You will sing along badly to the CD in the car and not care if you're out of tune.

3. Cleanliness will become mutually important (you'll shower together, clean teeth at the sink together, cut each other's toenails, he'll watch you shave your legs etc.).

4. You won't worry about matching underwear anymore.

5. You'll send him to the shops for tampons – and he'll go.

6. He'll hold your hair back when you're being sick.

7. You'll rub his back when he's being sick.

8. You'll eat off each other's plates (but not in pukey-couple way – no feeding each other like choo-choo trains).

9. He admits his soft spot for David Beckham (in an almost gay way).

10. You dance around your lounge together without being drunk.

11. You have unforgiving sex in broad daylight and not care if you've shaved or not.

12. You wake up to find him looking at you.

13. You sniff his clothes when he's not with you.

14. You talk about what you're doing on New Year's Eve – together.

15. He asks you to check his text messages (he's not scared about lurking exes or new blood).

16. You laugh at the same jokes.

17. He cries at the ending of a film and lets you pass him a tissue.

18. You talk about your school days.

19. You discuss where your parents went right and where they went wrong.

20. Sometimes you just have to kiss each other for hours and you don't know why.

Is it love?

If you have done at least ten of the above, think about him at least 102 times a day, can't even remember what your ex-boyfriends look like and have started naming future (imaginary) children, you got it bad. This is the real thing. 'Even Better Than the Real Thing', according to Bono.

How to say: 'I love you' without cringing

Beware of the man who tells you he loves you very early on in your dating diary. He may fall in love easily, say it to everyone he meets (even the postman) and not take it as seriously as you do. Don't read too much into it and don't feel you have to say it back.

Make sure you know what you're doing when you tell someone you love him or her. This is the turning point. There's no going back... he'll know how you feel, he'll be forced to respond and once it's out in the open, your relationship will pick up a gear.

The coward's way

◆ Get drunk and slur, or shout: 'I love you, I do. You're friggin' gorgeous. Do ya lurve me? Well, come on...do ya? Do ya? Ya do? Ya hoo!'

◆ Write lots of love, much love, I love you or all my love when you sign off a note.

◆ Punch him jokingly and say 'Oh I do love you, you're so funny!'

The love expert's way

Look him in the eye, tell him why he's special and then say loudly and clearly, 'I love you.'

How he responds shouldn't be taken to heart. As long as he doesn't spontaneously vomit, cry or run away, feel good about being honest. If he says it back with a smile, perfect. If he says thank you, he's flattered. If he doesn't say anything but gives you a cuddle, he's slightly embarrassed but thinks you're sweet. If he laughs kindly, laugh too and play it down.

Of course most modern girls choose the drunken, oops-I-don't-know-what-I'm-saying-me routine. This is fine. Saying I love you is a scary thing, as David Cassidy will testify. If you're drunk, he is likely to be drunk too, so it will be easier for him to respond. Once those three words are out there, it will get easier and easier to say them until you can't speak, text, email, sign without them coming into every correspondence at least twice. My husband and I got so fed up with our own mushiness after four months of dating, we set up a secret whispered language to cut down on the cringe factor. He would mouth, 'Two and a half pee?' and I would silently respond, 'Colourful.' Try it and you'll get the gist. This code is also fun to practise on complete strangers in a bar, or nightclub. They will run away faster than the wind so don't do it to anyone you quite fancy.

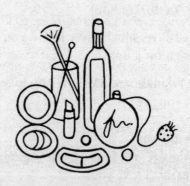

> **HANNAH,** 25
>
> ❝ I told my boyfriend I loved him by accident. We'd just had a major argument. I'd never been so angry with anyone in my whole life... I wanted to punch his lights out. But instead I sort of barked, screamed, and screeched like a mad lady: 'And to think I thought I was in love with you, you self-centred prick.' This really shut him up. He wrestled me to the floor and covered me in kisses. I told him I'd changed my mind and I now hated him but he didn't believe me. Which is just as well really because we've now got a one-year-old and are very much in love. ❞

The seven stages of love

After dating for a few months, you think the emotional battles are over and then a whole new pack of emotions and insecurities come and smack you round the face. Blimey, relationships are difficult. Love is a roller coaster.

1. Flirting. You're like a peacock and peahen prowling around each other, showing your best side and being constantly gorgeous, witty, and tempting.

2. Shagging. You haven't got time to get to know each other – apart from physically. This is fun.

3. Shyness. The physical side of things is now joined by the emotional. You become a bundle of nerves and questions run around your head.

4. Love. You've told each other how you feel. You are joined at the hip, your friends are starting to get annoyed and your mothers are starting to buy hats.

5. Arguments. He's not perfect? Well, no one told you.

6. Friendship. He really knows more about you than anyone else. He's your emergency number. You'd rather go to the cinema with him than anyone else.

7. Contentment. You've settled into a routine of stability and happiness. Sounds boring? It isn't. You've just stopped playing games – which means you've got more time to spend on the good stuff like shagging, laughing, seeing friends, decorating, going on holiday etc.

Being a non-sad, smug couple

There's nothing worse than being one of those icky, hands-everywhere couples so don't become one. Everyone (well, nearly) will be pleased you've met such a nice chap but they don't want his dimensions rammed down their throats. Neither do they want to invite you over for dinner and then be forced to make small talk while you snog each other all night. It's rude and the invites will dry up. The whole world isn't in love. You're the lucky ones. Keep it to yourselves.

NB Public displays of affection. People do assume – rightly or wrongly – that the old adage 'she doth protest too much' can be applied to couples that are too full on in public. What are they really like when the theatrics calm down?

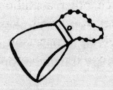

Maintain your own identity

Even if he has quickly replaced other interests in your life, pretend to still be your own person. Force yourself to go out on your own, with family, with friends or colleagues. You'll have fun when you do. Don't let the old you disappear. He fell in love with the old you so she must be a wonderful person. Fingers crossed things won't go wrong but if they do you need to have a life to go back to. Don't give up your interests for him. Just make more room for everything by ditching the boring things (watching all the soaps, obsessing over bathroom cleanliness or being a gym addict).

Keeping the dream alive

Dating is a difficult – and dangerous – process. You're putting your heart (and your sanity) on the line. But if it weren't worth the risk, falling in love wouldn't be the subject of so many songs, films and books. Love really does lift us all up where we belong.

So what do you do with love when you've got it? Well, if your dating has gone successfully (you've deduced he's not a murderer, pest or pervert), you can pass this book on to a friend and think about spending the rest of your days in blissful companionship.

But remember, the high you get when you first start dating someone doesn't last forever. Relationships get harder and harder to maintain, keep fresh and stay true. But everything is rescue-able. Where love is concerned, you deserve to give each other a million chances. If you still fancy him, he makes you laugh, you can't resist giving his hair a ruffle and he's the first person you want to call when you've got good or bad news – your dating days are over... for a while at least.

Secrets of Success

◆ Keep the television out of the bedroom – it will kill your sex life.

◆ Tell him off if he keeps referring to joint things as 'mine' or things you do together as 'when I'. He's either in relationship denial or a self-centred fool, so pull him up on it or find out which one of the above is the problem.

◆ Admit you need breathing space. Enjoy your own company or disappear in the bathroom for two hours rather than hanging around together and picking at each other until you have an argument.

◆ Honesty isn't always the best policy. You want to remain an Aphrodite-like figure in his eyes, a vision of loveliness for him to worship. Don't share too much – burping, gurning and sharing sexploit tales with his mates on your first meeting will leave him more willing to fight you than fancy you.

◆ If his friend hits on you, that's the mate's problem – not his. Do tell your partner if you think you haven't made yourself clear enough to the creep. But leave him out of it if you can. It

will cause arguments, as he will be forced to choose one of you over the other. Of course you are more fabulous than his sleazy buddy but they may have been friends a long time.

◆ Even when he's driving you mad, don't be tempted to snoop through his private belongings, searching for evidence of misdemeanours. Unless you have worthy suspicions of wrongdoings, calm down Little Miss Nosy. You wouldn't like him to read your old diaries now, would you?

◆ Most men love their mothers unconditionally; so don't even try to change his mind. He'll dump you before he dumps her – even if she is a nightmare. There's no such thing as a perfect family – he probably finds yours equally annoying – so try to connect on some level... even if it means being enthusiastic over his shopaholic mother's shoe collection. Men are slightly more objective about siblings, but don't do imitations or comment on his sister's weight, moustache, or lack of brain.

◆ If some of your friends have made derogatory comments about him, don't let him in on them. He'll get hurt, you'll defend them, he'll slag them off, you'll fight... you'll finish? To be honest, unless he is a complete loser and you're momentarily blinded by love, they should keep their gobs shut anyway.

◆ Perhaps the biggest argument-inciter is acknowledging you fancy someone else – even if it's just 'that bloke off the telly', he'll get jealous. And what are you trying to achieve? Leave lusting after others out until you've been together six months, the sex has diminished to twice a week (at weekends) and he's showed more than a passing interest in Heather Graham.

◆ If you accidentally (drunkenly) snog someone during your 'get together' period, don't tell him. At least, not until you've weighed up what it means to you. If it really was a tongue-fiddler shortly before puking in pub toilets (and you regret it and never want to do it again), don't tell him. He may think it's more serious than it was, he'll call you a few names and you'll argue your point for hours until he dumps you... unless you stay together with a massive trust issue.

◆ Sometimes arguing is healthy – but not in front of others (you'll be crossed off everyone's invitation list). Making up is definitely healthy – but not in front of others. Snogging after squabbling turns most people's stomachs.

◆ Do not get pregnant to trap a man. Modern girls know how to use contraception. We are smart – we know how to manage our bodies. Remember to check your pill packet if you have been ill or on antibiotics etc. Everyone has accidents but deliberately getting pregnant will not make him love you any more (probably even less) and it's not fair on the baby. Decide to have a child together – or make him fully aware you intend to have a child and tell him the options.

◆ You can be in love and still fancy other people. Don't feel guilty. It means you've still got blood rushing around your body... and everyone loves a flirt – it may even spark up you sex life at home. Fantasies are free.

◆ Even people who frown upon infidelity can find themselves in difficult situations which test their highest principles. No one knows how he or she'll cope with an unfaithful partner until it happens to him or her. Should you stay or should you go? Once bitten, twice shy or better the devil you know. Some people are serial philanderers. Others have genuinely fallen in love with someone else, or are searching for something to fill the void, or need attention after a period of neglect. Decide what's best for you. Listen to others' opinions but rely on your instincts when making the final decision.

◆ Don't say I love you after three dates.

◆ Don't scream if he doesn't say I love you straight back at you. It might have been a shock, he might not feel it yet (at least he's honest) or he may be waiting for more romantic surroundings to say it in.

◆ Likewise, don't feel forced to return the compliment if you don't mean it. Wait until you do.

◆ Don't get engaged unless it's to get married. That's what an engagement means – it's not a chance to get a free diamond and a toaster from your grandma.

◆ Don't get engaged unless you're as sure as you can be that it's the right thing to do. Sounds silly but it's easy to get carried away with the idea of a big dress and a party. But it's more than a wedding, it's a marriage... and that means a massive sharing of responsibility, money and future. Think carefully. Divorces are common, but painful, expensive and tiring.

◆ Some things are too intimate and should be avoided even when you are truly in love. I'm thinking golden showers, anything involving animals and letting him pluck your bikini line. No.

◆ Don't get too depressed if your Mr Perfect turns out to be no such thing. Most men aren't. Handle it or get fishing.

◆ Don't let anyone give you a timeline. If you want to move in together after three months, do it. Just beware you might not know each other very well yet. If you get married within a year, fine. Don't feel you have to conform to society's expectations, or 'do things properly'. Some of the longest, loveliest relationships have been sealed after a courtship of six months.

◆ Swallow your pride. If you love him, fight to the end and hang the consequences. A modern girl must always use her head – but her heart should play a big part too.

◆ Enjoy it. There's nothing to beat waking up next to your soul mate.

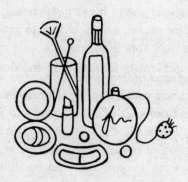

Further Reading

Biddulph, Steve and Biddulph, Shaaron, *How Love Works*, HarperCollins, 2000

Browne, Joy (Dr), *Dating For Dummies*, Running Press Miniature Editions, 2000

Cox, Tracey, *Hot Sex*, Corgi, 1999

Daily, Lisa, *Stop Getting Dumped*, Plume Books, 2002

Fein, Ellen and Schneider, Sherrie, *The Rules for Online Dating*, Pocket Books, 2002

Gray, John, *Men are from Mars, Women are from Venus*, HarperCollins, 2002

Lewis, Cherry, *The Dating Game*, Cambridge University Press, 2002

McGraw, Phillip C., *Relationship Rescue*, Vermilion, 2002

Nicholls, Anne, *Make Love Work for You*, Piatkus, 2002

Tysoe, Maryon, *The Good Relationship Guide*, Piatkus, 1997

Index